Align Your Spirit, Soul & Body
to Reach Total Health

Align Your Spirit, Soul & Body to Reach Total Health

By C.O. Aguirre

Align Your Spirit, Soul & Body
to Reach Total Health

Written by C.O. Aguirre.

First edition. July 4, 2020.

Copyright © 2020 C.O. Aguirre.

ISBN- 978-1-7353587-0-3

In honor of my mother, who taught me

the meaning of endurance.

Contents

About the Cover

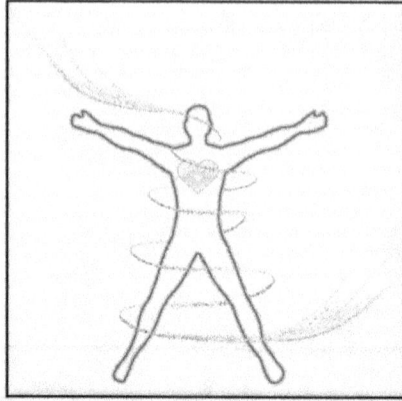

Someone asked me what the symbolism behind the book cover is. For those inquiring minds, here is the meaning of it:

I created the body figure based on the Vitruvian Man by Leonardo DaVinci that represents the ideal human body proportions. DaVinci explained that his drawing was part work of mathematics, part work of art signifying how everything connects to everything in the universe.

This book supports DaVinci's belief and honors it by putting the human figure on the cover. The rest of the symbolism you will have to discover by reading the book.

Happy reading!

Chapter 1

C.O. Aguirre

Why I Wrote this Book

I am delighted to present to you this book about total health. The body is not a solo unit but a part of three. Our body, soul, and spirit are connected and dependent on each other for survival. So, when we talk about total health, we must also address how to keep our spirit and soul in top shape.

The concept of spiritual health came to me when I found myself diagnosed with cancer. I knew that I wasn't ready to face the end of my life on earth, but I also understood that there was something missing in my concept of health. That's when I decided to gather all experience and knowledge I had about healing in my spirit, soul and body, even though the thought of it was very overwhelming.

In my search for that spiritual health, and to figure out what was missing, I took the point of view of a spiritual healer. I am not a shaman. And I am not a medical therapist. The term spiritual healer is based on the connection and knowledge I have of the Light from a spiritual and scientific point of view.

The beginning of my days as a healer started when my parents introduced me to religion as a kid. Most importantly, my mother taught me to pray for the sick. She was a woman who went beyond religion and understood life to be more than just the physical world. She believed the spiritual dimension was the ruler of our world.

Once I went to college and became independent, I left home and left religion behind. I did not think I needed them. Science was more appealing to me and I became fascinated by it.

Getting rid of the religious side of me left me with no outlet to deal with the things that had no explanation outside the devout world. So, I came back to religion after a series of big losses in my life. At that time, I was hungry to know the explanations about why "bad things" happened to me. I also became a chaplain and started to volunteer praying for the sick. I absorbed everything I could. I got to the point where religion didn't have all the answers or the answers I received, did not sync well with my spirit.

I became emotionally drained from conflicting information coming my way and nobody seemed to have satisfying answers as to what was the right or wrong way to look at things. I decided to expand my spiritual search into other religions and dogmas to see if they had an answer.

I can truly say that every faith that I explored was amazing in its own way. All of them had invaluable knowledge. But those nagging questions about conflicting information would not go away. Only one thing was clear to me – the Light. That higher being was real because I could feel it thriving within me when I had peace, hope, or love. But religious traditions would limit that energy and put it in a box full of conflicting knowledge.

In my search to find what synced with my spirit, I expanded my quest beyond the dogmas of the world. I was totally surprised when the answers to my questions came from a place I would have never imagined – science. Yes, science, the one place that does not support the idea of a spiritual world or a god, became the basis for my spiritual beliefs. What was surprising was that from quantum physics, to genetics, to biology, to chemistry, all roads seem to lead to the Light, that higher being that was the center of my spirituality. I discovered that the Light manifested in science through this electromagnetic vibration that exists everywhere and is the essence of all matter.

My discovery of science syncing with spirituality became more evident. I understood that hope, peace, and love were not just emotions or states of mind that people could have. They were sources of positive energy that healed the body and science backed it up. My experience as a chaplain and my ten plus years praying for the sick solidified my perspective as a "spiritual healer."

Armed with my experiences, I embarked on my healing journey. I always thought of health only in a physical aspect. I was not aware of what mental health was until I experienced major losses. During that time in my life, I couldn't get out of that "blue" state of mind. I thought it would just go away on its own and eventually I would go back to my old self. But time did not heal me. In fact, my mental health started to have an adverse effect on me. That's when I decided to learn about issues like depression, anxiety, PTSD, and behavioral concerns. I wanted to know what was happening to me. Science calls these conditions mental health issues. I prefer to call them soul ailments because my emotions, decision making, and awareness became cloudy.

When I use the word "soul," I do not use it in reference to "soul mates" or the immortal side of a human being that goes to heaven, as some religions teach. Soul in this book has a unique definition. I call "soul" the three functions that make the body run: consciousness or mind, emotions and decision making. I explain all concepts in the chapters ahead.

My desire to know more about soul ailments took me on a healing journey where I met my higher being that I called the Light. The source of all positive energy is the Light. Becoming aware of the Light changed my life and the way I looked at it. There have been times when the pain I felt was excruciating and

I just wanted to "disappear." And the more I battled with life, the keener my connection with the Light became. I expected that my knowledge and connection with the Light would make the pain go away. And for a time, it did. But then, the emotional pain started to manifest in physical pain and illness. I didn't know that I had certain behaviors that were opening the door for me to become ill in my soul, spirit and body.

Little by little, my body started to break down. There were times when my body would get stronger because I would seek physical fitness, but those moments of health clarity started to dissipate because I wasn't taking care of the root problem – my spiritual health.

I knew deep inside that something needed to change because despite my efforts, I couldn't keep my peace of mind. In my search to know how I could get healthy, I immersed myself in a few dogmas and they were very helpful. I learned to meditate, to pray, to connect with the Light and the universe. I learned about how the world came to be, why contrition was a need and the path to have purpose in life. I learned about enlightenment, peace and morality. But spiritual health was not very clear. I do not recall anybody speaking to me about spiritual health or where to obtain the keys to total health.

Going through my cancer treatment, I comprehended the journey of so many people who suffer from it. The fear of the unknown and the loneliness can be overwhelming. Then, I realized that thanks to the Light, I overcame the fear and became encouraged that things would be OK. I wrote a list of things I wanted to change in my daily routine and a list of spiritual principles that I wanted to practice. This is when I knew I came up with a health program that was helping me in my spirit, soul and body. This was a program that helped me seek for total health.

Having my own health program was very encouraging and solidified my connection with the Light. I was in the middle of writing the book and still not sure if I should publish it, and then COVID-19 hit the world. I knew right then that my experience would benefit those looking for answers beyond science, the medical community and religion. When fear takes over the body, soul and spirit, a jolt of trust is needed to move forward. I have learned about this while being a spiritual healer.

I explain spirituality, positive energy, the sources of positive energy and a daily program to follow to keep the spirit, soul, and body in fit condition.

This book also explains the three parts of a human being that need healing in order to have total health. The first one is the human spirit, the second one is mental health and the third one is body fitness.

But what is your spirit? How can you recognize it? And how do you take care of it? This book will look at the spirit and the spiritual world not from a religious point of view, but from a look into quantum physics, chemistry, and genetics.

This book also explains from a spiritual and scientific point of view how to get in touch with your spirit and how to keep it healthy. It will teach you how to help with spiritual illnesses and guard your soul and body from getting ill and staying healthy.

I want to make sure to emphasize that the purpose of this book is not to replace medical treatment – it's exactly the opposite. Medical help is irreplaceable and spiritual help is a necessity. We should not ignore nor delay seeking help from either source.

I especially present this book to people struggling with health issues. Enduring illness for long periods of time takes a toll on a person's positive outlook. The uncertainty of the future, seeing the body deteriorate, feeling detached from the world, having a sense of loss – all these states of mind are hard to deal with on top of the pain that a person may be experiencing. I went through all of them and fought hard to find a way to deal with them and then wrote this book about it.

My answers in this book came from the connection I developed with the Light. Immersing in the Light's positive energy brought me back to life in every sense of the word. This is what I want to share with you, yes, you, the person who has a heavy load on his/her shoulders and needs help. This is for you…. from my heart to yours.

Chapter 2

C.O. Aguirre

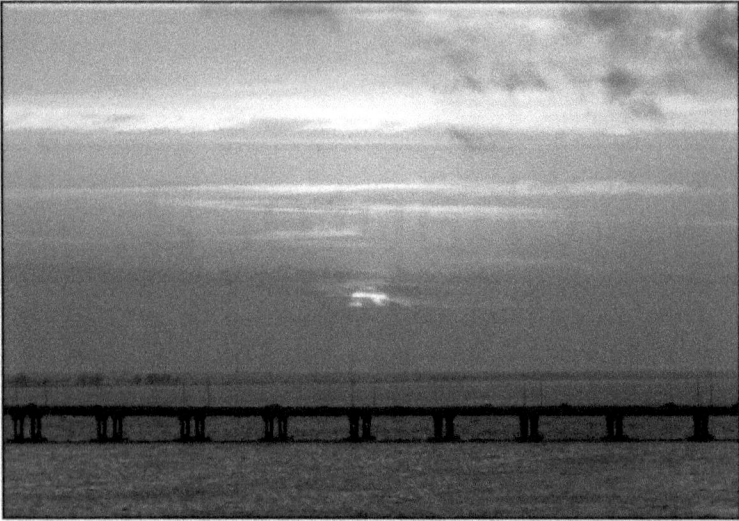

The Signs of Positive Energy Depletion

B efore I talk about what is the energy that boosts the spirit and the soul, I want to talk about the depletion of positive energy and its effects on the body.

Positive energy is like recharging the battery of the human spirit. When the battery is fully charged, the soul and the body have what they need to function properly. When the battery gets low, we start to lose hope and peace. Life starts to feel like it's too heavy to handle. This is a sign that we cannot ignore.

When I was a teenager, my dad died in a car accident. I understand now that my mind couldn't completely understand what was happening and the ramification of my loss. And even though I was around people who could counsel me how to deal with loss, I don't think anybody did. My mom was trying to deal with her own emotions. She was pregnant with my youngest sister. I understand now that the responsibility of going from housewife to breadwinner didn't leave her enough time to take care of herself and even less to make sure all her children were coping with the loss of my dad.

When I left home to go to college, I felt another great loss in my life. I reacted similarly to the way I did when I lost my dad. Even though it was a great event happening in my life, I was also losing my culture, my life and my family. It was a very hard step for me.

The third time I felt like the foundation of my life was shaken was when I was laid-off from my job after college. I tried to brush it off my shoulder just like I did before, but I couldn't. This was the first time I noticed what happened to me every time I felt like the changes in the foundation of my life shook "my future." I felt a spiritual detachment that brought emotional and spiritual pain. They manifested like strong emotions of loss, absence, and misplacement.

The interesting part of going through these emotions was that the more they happened to me, the less I believed I was capable to overcome. This was a sign of my spiritual battery getting low.

The following is a list of circumstances that deplete the spiritual battery, disconnecting the human spirit to the source of life, the Light: pain, suffering and loss. Let's look at them closely.

Pain

Most people associate the word pain to physical pain. The medical community classifies pain as acute and chronic. Acute pain comes from injury and may not last a long time. Chronic pain lasts for long periods of time and its source may be known or unknown. This is the kind of pain that debilitates a person and little by little corrodes and diminishes the positive outlook in a person.

In my case, I know pain debilitated me because when I saw that no matter what treatments I received, the pain wouldn't go away, I became frustrated and hopeless. I wanted to believe that everything would be OK, but it was like the pain had more endurance than me. At the end of the day, I would lose the battle of believing that I would eventually go back to being me. After a while, I was not just hopeless but angry.

When I volunteered as a chaplain, I saw the same feelings in people I prayed for who had chronic pain. The battle is fierce and real. The cheerful person inside would get smaller and smaller and their positive outlook in life would disappear. Chronic pain will deplete a person's desire to participate in life because of the limitations it puts on a person. This type of pain is for sure a destroyer of the positive energy in a person.

Suffering

When I think of the word suffering, I immediately think about physical pain. And yes, suffering encompasses physical pain, but it also touches the realm of emotions in the soul like a feeling of agony or misery.

There is also such a thing as misery in the spirit. An example of spiritual suffering is the struggle that all human beings experience at some point in their life where a person cannot control the outcome of life. A person who has struggled with life understands that despite their best effort, life brings losses. There is no prediction when or how they will occur.

That agony of not being able to have control can for sure shake the foundations of a person's belief system. Not being able to know or to trust the unknown future of my loved ones is a suffering that starts in the spirit because that's where the knowledge resides about my soul and my body.

Not being able to stop the pain, the mind gets affected. This unrest manifesting as suffering and pain in the spirit, slowly but surely affects the soul's mental health. The suffering can even reflect in the body as physical pain. Going through losses in life opens a person's eyes about how little control we have on life. When the answers cannot come from people, we tend to look into the spiritual realm. This is why religions have existed from the beginning of time. They all offer an answer to the question of suffering.

I do not remember being a happy child or being overly happy as an adult. Even though I have achieved a lot of success, it has not translated into my mind as happiness. This unhappiness comes from that place in my mind where I have a tendency to suffer. I used to focus on things I wanted to have but couldn't or the rejection I felt from people. This tendency, I understand now, had made me partial to feel sad about my life in general. I think this "state of unhappiness" came as a result of many things that happened in my childhood. I learned not to trust, to detach myself from others and to see the glass as "half empty" instead of "half full." I became predisposed to see my life as a painful experience instead of being grateful for it. I did not notice this until my suffering became unbearable.

Then, my counselor guided me into looking back and noticing that wherever I went, I did great things, but they did not bring me happiness. I expected people to notice my achievements and pat me on the back. When they didn't, I was easily discouraged, especially if the feedback came in the form of criticism and negative observations. It didn't matter how much success I achieved. I couldn't make me happy because what I was looking for was a connection, a button that I could click within me that made me happy, but I couldn't find that button. My efforts became null and the sadness in my heart just grew a little bigger each time.

The little piles of sadness became a mountain of sorrows. I did not lack a roof over my head or food on my table. In fact, I've been blessed to have all I needed. But it never occurred to me to be happy by looking at these things. I could only think of the many things life would not give me. I know I sound like a spoiled brat that was never satisfied, but I can assure you that this angst didn't have anything to do with me being a spoiled child. This pain was real. It felt like a void within me and I looked everywhere to find the missing part of the puzzle. And I tried and tried and tried, but the more I tried, the more lost I felt.

I did not know how to heal this pain, so I did nothing. Letting the pain grow was a doorway I open to spill my positive energy.

Loss

The impact of losing someone or something reminds us the fact that we are not in control. Having to face this can produce fear, anxiety, stress, hopelessness, and other emotions that are gut wrenching and painful experiences. The grief caused by the death of a loved one can be the crossroads that changes the course of our life. Even when we feel that our life stopped when we lost that special person, being stuck in that moment of sorrow can affect the rest of our life.

The loss of my mother was that crossroads for me. In so many ways, it wasn't just her person that I mourned. It was a series of wishes and hopes that never came to be. It took me years to come to peace with all those little parts of my heart to be identified and reconstructed.

Reflecting on the death of my mom, I look back at our relationship. I remember a strict person who always expected my best performance. When I didn't perform up to par, which was usually always, I would be deprived of the praise that I desperately wanted. As a child, I thought that praise was a sign of love. Later in life, I realized that she showed love in a different way. Still, understanding did not stop my heart from desiring her praise. It didn't help either that my role model for a mother were the moms I saw on TV. Besides the praise, I wanted my mother to say and do the things I saw the TV moms do, where she would love me just as I was.

When my mom died, the sorrow I felt was overwhelming. It took me years to go through the five stages of grief. And after almost 10 years, sometimes I still feel that sorrow deep in my gut. I understand now that her loss was so intense because I was mourning the hope that someday, she would love me just the way I thought a mother would love a child. Her death killed that hope and coming to terms with this loss took me years.

Loss is another gate in our spirit that when it opens, it causes a leak in our positive energy. If left unattended, it can turn into mental health issues or even manifest in physical illness.

The effects of negative energy feeding my pain

We all have those moments in life when we come face to face with fear. The impact is so overwhelming and painful that the aftermath lasts a lifetime. One of these moments for me was the COVID 19 pandemic. Being confined at home by the threat of a virus that shrank the world economy and took the life of so many people paralyzed me for a while.

The sudden realization that we are not in control brings us down to our knees. Our first reaction is to fight back, but how can we fight the invisible and unknown? We do all we can to ensure we will not be defeated and even when we buy enough hand sanitizer to last a lifetime, we realize this is not enough to win the war.

When we feel defeat at our door and the strength leaves us, we realize we must find a way to survive. It is at this crossroads that we make a decision that changes our life. A few years back, my therapist said it the best way, "The choice is love or fear. What will you choose?"

Love is the highest source of positive energy. Love gives me the strength and wisdom to fight back in a way that edifies and brings hope not just to me but people around me. Love brings allies to my team. Love will give me the creativity needed to survive.

But if we choose fear, the picture becomes quite different. We may not realize it when we make the decision, but our future becomes bleak.

I know about what happens when choosing fear because I had to go through a very rough patch in my life. I didn't know at the time what I was choosing or the consequences of my decisions. I just reacted to the events happening in my life. I ended up depleted of my positive energy and sick. The following are examples of how fear ravaged my life.

Loneliness

Someone told me once that I was a social butterfly. I never saw myself that way, but I can see that now. But before I started on my healing journey, I felt lonely and abandoned. This loneliness had nothing to do with me being alone or having difficulty doing things on my own or being in a quarantine. I have never been afraid of approaching a person or talking to strangers. In fact, if I could count the number of people I have gotten along with, I can say that I am indeed a social butterfly. But when I felt alone, I certainly did not feel or see myself like I was approachable or liked by people.

This loneliness was a perception of the mind and a feeling in the pit of my stomach that took me to isolation. It was not a feeling that I felt 24/7. But, when it would strike, that feeling removed me from social circles, friends, and family. I do not know when it started but what I know is that loneliness feels like a flood that inundated every single area of my life and detached me from my life.

At first, loneliness only made its presence felt when I came home in the evening and I would sit at home wishing someone was around. Little by little, it grew as if I started to be removed from my own mind and the feeling would take over my mind and emotions. It became like an obsession that I couldn't get rid of. I would go to have a drink after work with co-workers and I felt uncomfortable. Or I would go volunteer, as I would twice a week, and I felt like a misfit. Then, it took over my work. I felt like I did not want to talk to anyone around me because I felt that nobody understood me. Being around my family during the holidays was the straw that broke the camel's back. It was so painful and solitary because I felt judged for not meeting my family's expectations.

I found myself trapped in a box where I wanted to reach out, but it was too painful to even try because I felt I did not belong outside the box anymore. It was as if I wanted to protect myself from the judgement of the world. I wanted with all my heart to be accepted but I felt nobody wanted to be inclusive. I knew something needed to change but it never occurred to me that the change started with me.

I wanted the world to change and make me feel like I belonged. I knew nobody would go out of their way to make me feel that way, so why bother getting out of the box? Then, I thought I could overcome this feeling of isolation by making myself attractive and charming. But I didn't have the strength to transform me in such a way because nothing I did worked. I felt trapped in a body of a loser who couldn't do what I needed to do to attract people to like me.

The truth of the matter was that I had no clue if people really wanted to reject me or not. I was the one judging myself and trying to get into a shape of a person that I thought would be pleasant to others. But that shape was not who I was. It was like wanting to fit into a dress that was 5 sizes smaller than mine. How could I fit in such a dress? It was impossible. Nonetheless, here I was trying to become a person that was not me and the more I tried, the more isolated and lonelier I became.

Being lonely was so painful, not because I was isolated but because I was afraid I wasn't made in the shape of people's liking. I felt I was not suitable to be around people. I was the first one rejecting and judging myself and taking myself out of the equation. I wanted to be around people and be accepted but I was afraid I would only get rejected. I wanted to be successful and popular and admired by people, but the fear of them not wanting to welcome me was stronger. It was really a total mess in my head, and I couldn't see what I was doing right or wrong because I was confused. This was one of the most perplexing moments in my life. I knew what I wanted, I tried everything under the sun to achieve it and ended up back in the box, sad, frustrated and lonely.

I used to ask myself, "How many times should I go out there and try to connect?" This became the question I started to ask myself. Have I not tried long enough to just let it go? The pain in my soul grew larger and larger and the agony became stronger. It was like loneliness had broken my two legs and now I was paralyzed on my journey in life. I started to doubt if life was worth all these crazy efforts.

I think my inability to connect and "perform" in society was the start of the next phase I encountered in my life journey. Life became a series of questions and it didn't matter what answers I gave; they never were good enough to satisfy the questions. This constant questioning became anxiety for me.

Anxiety

According to social science, anxiety is a form of fear. The way I experienced anxiety in the past was a mixture of fear and an urgency to find an answer that would ease my worries. It manifested when I started a project and I did not know if the outcome would be in my favor. It became a worry that would not stop and started to affect my health mentally and physically. It was like I put my mind in overdrive and I could not stop it from worrying.

Using the example of my mind as a computer, our mind searches for answers when we have a problem to solve. When our mind says, ask for advice, it means that we have to use the resources outside our mind to find the answer.

During this project, my anxiety felt like my mind was looking for answers and I couldn't find them within me, so I had to expand my search to other people. The thought of me having to trust people to get answers was overwhelming because I felt I couldn't trust them. I wanted to trust them, but I couldn't because I was afraid. In my mind they weren't trustworthy, and I knew I couldn't control the situation.

When my attempts to trust people and get assurance were not fulfilled, my mind became confused. I desperately wanted to feel safe, but my mind told me I couldn't. Then, my mind became a platform of statements of "what if." Every statement in my head was, "What if I do this?" but the more I asked, the less answers I got. And the more my mind rushed to conclusions, the more fear and anxiety became my safety net.

I am so grateful that anxiety is not a ruler of my mind anymore. But that doesn't mean that it doesn't try to sneak in here and there. When anxiety takes over my mind, it usually debilitates me, confuses me and destroys my ability to see that there is always a Light at the end of the tunnel.

I remember I got very anxious when I broke up with my first boyfriend. My family expected me to get married and have a family. I feared my mother's response and criticism for me not being able to please a man to stay with me. I didn't think she would understand that I broke up with him because I didn't feel like he was the man I wanted to spend the rest of my life with. He was the perfect man for what my family wanted but he was not what I needed in my life. For days I dreaded the thought of telling my mother. My anxiety would rise, and I would feel confused and incapacitated to speak or think when the thought of facing my mother came to mind.

To make a long story short, one Sunday evening, I prepared a list of things and reasons why I couldn't marry this man and I called my mother up. (Some were true, others exaggerated, and a couple were lies to make me seem like a victim – my mother definitely would not resist the desire to protect me from this horrible man). With a broken voice and in tears, I told her that I wasn't in a relationship anymore. She heard me and kept silent for a second. Then, she just muttered the word, "okay." Nothing else. When I hung up the phone, my anxiety disappeared.

This anxiety came back a few years later when I separated from my ex-husband which eventually led to divorce. I think I used to have a panic attack every day that I was supposed to tell my mother and I didn't. I was becoming the first woman in the family to get divorced and bring shame to the family. One Saturday evening I finally told my mother. Her response was, "Finally! That man was neurotic." I didn't know if I should have laughed or cried, but the relief I felt was indeed a miracle.

Even though I went through these experiences, I did not become aware of the lesson here: Anxiety is not the response that I need from my soul when I am worried and stressed about my circumstances. Anxiety does not give me the strength to feel empowered and assured. Anxiety is a tool that opens my heart to doubt my abilities, my confidence and my future. It wasn't until I started my healing journey that I realized I needed to ditch the anxiety program out of my mind.

Running away

I make friends easily and I never stop to think about how many real friends I have had in my life. I used to have trust issues. I had (and still have) a tendency to become friends with people and at the first sign I saw that I couldn't trust them, I just tossed them aside and kept on going with my life. I didn't know this was a form of running away. My therapist did a good job in highlighting how easy it was for me not to hold on to relationships, friends, jobs and pretty much everything. At work, when I didn't like the way I was treated, I would take a trip overseas. The new sights and experiences would appease me for a while but then my emotions would get the best of me when the same situation would present itself at work. I knew I had to deal with the emotions I had, but instead, I would just find another job in hopes that the situation would be different at the new job. I didn't know how to deal with conflict because my heart was full of fear. And not just any kind of fear – the fear of rejection, so my best strategy was to "run away."

I knew I couldn't run away forever so I found another way to appease the fears. That strategy became watching TV. My rationalizing was that it helped me relax and take the edge off. Sometimes I still do this, and I find myself sitting in front of the TV avoiding life.

Being in my health journey made me aware of this behavior. And just like me, I realize millions of people choose behaviors or substances to ease the edge of life. I want to use the metaphor of my mind being like a chess computer. Every time it loses; it finds a solution not to lose again. My mind is like this kind of computer. Every single emotion, trauma and pain that I go through, my soul/mind tries to find a solution for it. Sounds good, right? Not so great when I discovered a glitch. When I couldn't find the solution for my pain, I numbed it, which to me was better than taking action. What an interesting computer program! My mind has the power to take over my will when I am feeling frightful and I do not want to deal with life.

Being committed to my healing journey taught me that running away is painful because it causes me to not deal with the real issue and only postpone the inevitable. And dealing with the issue is painful because I have to learn to take the monsters out of the closet and learn to deal with conflict and stand up to fear.

I remember the first time I decided to confront my fears and speak up for myself. I was in tears in front of my boss asking why I was passed over for a promotion that I had earned fair and square. I knew she wasn't going to give me what I wanted but I also understood that in order to see myself differently I needed to say something. The agony I went through just imagining what I would say and how she would react was insufferable.

Many times, I asked myself why it was so painful. Why I couldn't stop crying. Instead of bringing me closure, it brought me shame, regret and the pain was stronger. It took many months before I decided to be "assertive" and speak up for myself. In fact, I had to change jobs to feel better about myself.

I understand now that running away is a sign of me not liking very much who I am. It wasn't that I had no value, but I couldn't see the value in me and that caused me pain. It wasn't like people were rejecting me, but I was rejecting myself before anyone else and that caused me pain. I used to think that I was running away from people because I didn't want them to hurt me. Now I understand that the one I was running away from was me. I did not know how to obtain self-esteem. And I didn't know how to stand up to that nagging voice inside me. That voice that said that I didn't have what it took to be me, to be successful, to be attractive, to be engaging, and to be accepted. I thought that voice was me and I just accepted what it said. Now I know this was the voice of self-loathing. It disguises as if it were my voice and beats me over with no mercy. Self-hatred gets its power from the fear of rejection I feel and they both try to destroy my identity.

I feel blessed that in my healing journey, I have learned that not all voices in my head using the "I" pronoun are me. I do not have to listen to any voice that causes me pain or tells me that I am not good enough. I do not have to pay attention to that voice that finds fault in all I do and judges me mercilessly. This is the voice that comes to steal who I am, to kill my identity and to destroy what I build. I thank the Light for helping me discover that this stinging, hurtful voice hiding inside me, is not me. I must not listen to it because there is no truth in it.

Today, I do not run away or numb the pain. Today, I love myself to the best of my abilities.

Anger

This is a very volatile emotion. It boils in the gut in a nano second and with a look or a word, I have the power to cut someone out of my life and/or manipulate them. Many people have hurt or murdered a person out of passion, meaning out of anger. We all have the capability of doing this in a moment of passion. Why? Because anger is one emotion that can become rage in a second. Rage takes away my self-control and it lashes back to the person who "injured" me as a pay back from the pain I am experiencing.

Anger is a healthy emotion that shows me when my boundaries have been trespassed but if I let it go unchecked, it can become rage and force me to be hostile against others in just a moment. How do I know when it becomes aggression? I know it when I feel a heat that rises in my belly and increases my heartbeat and blood pressure. It rationalizes my desire for revenge as necessary justice. But most of the time, when rage takes over my will, I won't even have a second to question what is happening to me.

In my healing journey, I noticed that my upbringing gave room to anger because I was taught that "good girls" do not speak back or argue with people. I felt trapped in my mind with these rules that were imposed on me. I could not defend myself when I felt someone was trespassing my boundaries or emotionally "injuring" me. Why couldn't I defend myself? Why should I let others step all over me? Not having a good answer for these questions, the negative energy accumulated in my mind. It would whisper in my ear that I was weak when I couldn't stand up for myself. I believe this voice was shame and self-hatred and listening to this voice allowed anger to give me the energy that I needed to defend myself and seek justice for myself.

I cannot tell you how many times I beat up myself, and judged myself harshly, for not being able to speak up for myself. The self-judgement came as a voice in my mind calling me a "loser." It felt so real and made me powerless every time I felt that voice coming. It made me become a passive aggressive responder. I didn't want to explode but I did because in my mind people were hurting me. I felt that they disregarded me and wouldn't consider my feelings. These assumptions I created in my mind made me feel like a loser because I couldn't stop people from walking all over me. These thoughts would not leave me alone and I would lash out in the most inappropriate places and occasions.

When I think back about why I got upset, I have to point out to those assumptions and judgements I made in my mind. I believed them to be real. I wanted so badly to find respect and validation, but I was the first one not to give it to me. This made my world come crashing down. All I wanted was for people to pay for the injury caused against me.

The worst part about anger for me was that surprisingly when I got even, there was no satisfaction. I understood later in my healing journey that my anger and my desire to get even would not fix my desire for revenge because what really bothered me was that nagging "voice" in my head that called me names and judged me. That was really the issue.

The betrayal, the injury, the pain I felt could not compare to the injury I was causing myself. I understood later on that this was the voice of self-hatred fueled by fear and disguised as my voice. This voice would speak to me using the "I" pronoun, it would sound like me, and because of those reasons I thought it was true.

Self-hatred injected a lot of anger in my life. This anger made me miserable. It also stole the meaning of my life and destroyed my trust in myself. It even made me crazy. During my outbursts of anger, I would lose the perception of reality. Anger injects this volatile energy that may be perceived as empowerment. It is an emotion that feels like it encourages me to find justice. But in reality, it's an explosion that destroys anybody around me, including me. It leaves me full of shame and guilt, and with no desire to live after I realize what I have done. This explosion is fuel by the fear behind all my expectations going on in my head at the time of the outburst. Anger is the most dangerous emotion if left unattended. The fear attached to it will destroy everyone around me, especially me.

Expectations

Someone said to me that expectations are premeditated resentments. I didn't understand this until I started to see my therapist. When people didn't do as I expected, I would get mad and develop feelings of resentment towards them. I did not understand this process in my mind, and it was not evident to me until I worked on a project at work. I created a new business model for a client to make more money for the company. I just assumed that this would be my ticket to have a promotion and make more money. They ended up giving the position to a girl who became involved with the VP of the company. Needless to say, I got angry and went to speak to my boss. The explanation that my boss gave me was that the other girl had negotiating skills that I didn't.

I stayed at that job for one more year. During that time, the girl did not understand the system I created and always came to me asking for help. After ten months of doing this, she decided to leave the office in the United States and went back to the Canada office. When she left, my boss gave me her duties without a raise or a promotion. I once again fixed the system, proposed changes to the client and was successful to create a new model that would make my company more money. And just like the first time, my expectations were my demise. But instead of recognizing the negative energy that was killing me, my focus was on the expectations that didn't come to pass. I know that my attitude was an issue because I definitely acted like I was entitled to that promotion and raise. I don't know if I had shown a different attitude the outcome would have been different. I ended up changing jobs. Unfortunately, I did not leave behind my expectant and entitled attitude. It hurt me just as much in my next job.

Expectations are like a self-fulling prophecy based on fear that will always steal the best of us. The fear behind it says: "I am going to judge myself harshly and will be angry with the world because they failed to validate me and to recognize my worth." When in fact, the Light is the only one who can precisely validate me and tell me my worth because I am a little fragment of the Light. Nobody else has any idea or the capability to see what is inside of me.

Unfulfilled expectations are open doors for negative energy to come in and steal in exchange of filling us up with resentment (anger). This type of negative energy is bad for our health. According to studies, resentment is the kind of anger that keeps you up at night causing tremendous stress on the body. This type of anger sits in the gut and gets internalized, eating you up from the inside out. If left unattended, this kind of anger leads to anxiety and depression.

"But how can this feeling be wrong? All I want is justice," says the resentment voice in our head. Deep inside, we may be aware that anger is the cause for insomnia and anxiety. But if we let it go, we might feel that we are weak, and people could walk all over us because they did us wrong and we could not get justice for ourselves.

The truth of the matter is that the resentment voice infusing negative energy in us is like a vampire. It sucks all the good energy, creativity, and ideas out of us and then sets us up for failure so it can make a dwelling in our body. And while the resentment is in our gut, we lose perspective of reality because we are too angry to act like a civilized person, and people respond to this aggression by ignoring the good we have done.

I am very grateful for my healing journey and to the Light for finding gratitude, an option I found to exercise instead of resentment. It really changed my life. I talk about it in the coming chapters so stay tuned.

I see no reason for my life

I think at some point or another in our life, we wonder what the point of living is. When we are lacking love and validation of our existence, we often wonder what the purpose of our life is. Why live at all when nothing seems to go our way?

Why live? These were the words I told my friend when I separated from my ex-husband. This was a time when my hopes sort of died and I found myself hopeless. We all go through these periods when the loss is such that it takes away our dearest dreams, so we feel like we have no purpose in life anymore. It took me about 6 months to get out of this funk after my divorce. But the lessons that I learned were absolutely invaluable.

First lesson I learned about depression was that it cannot be ignored. If I fall and break my arm, there is no question in my mind that the next thing I need to do is go to the ER and get a cast. Unfortunately, with mental conditions there is still the myth that people will think we are "crazy," so we need to hide it. The reality is that those thoughts that tell you that looks and appearance are more important than your mental health, are wrong. You are important and your life matters. If you are feeling sad, hopeless, or confused and you do not know how to get out of this funk, you must seek help.

When it happened to me, I sought help with a counselor. I was so grateful that my time spent in therapy helped me understand that I was not the only one mourning the loss of divorce. It was at this time in my life when I first learned about support groups. I met several people who became life-time friends. In my first support group I learned about suffering and how fragile life can be after a painful event.

The second thing I learned was that my desire to change my circumstances back to where I liked it only made me very angry because that was impossible. I wanted to go back to that time I was happy and could not, so I became helpless and hopeless. It was a dreadful feeling to not have the desire to pick myself up from the floor. My ex-husband was my best friend, my support, my village and all of a sudden, I had nothing. I kept asking in my mind: "Why can I not have what so many people have?" I wasn't asking to have a billionaire husband, all I wanted was the guy that I fell in love with back into my life; that perky and chivalrous guy just like the first time I met him. Not being able to control my life made me angry. Letting go and moving on were not a cliché anymore. Those words saved me from myself.

Third thing I learned was that not letting go of the past extended my depression and my desire not to be around. I used to say, "What is the purpose of life if I cannot get what I want? Why bother fighting for a life I don't want?" Again, the words, "letting go" and "moving on" saved my life.

But the negative attitude was giving me something I didn't want to give up. This addictive energy made me sassy, sarcastic and funny. It was all good and great, but it wasn't me and it wasn't feeding my spirit. I was becoming this person who wrapped herself in negativity and people liked it, so I just kept the facade going, knowing that deep inside I was dying slowly. I didn't want anybody to enter into that room of my life because asking for help meant I had to let go of the things that people admired in me. Eventually I had the courage to find my worth and I was able to let it go and move on.

The fourth thing I learned was that by having this negative energy I was starving my spirit of positive energy and feeding it with three monsters: shame, guilt, and self-hatred. They all came out of my mouth in the form of sarcasm. I thought people admired and enjoyed in me this sarcasm; it became too much and too dark and people stopped wanting to be around me.

One day at my support group meeting, someone called me out about my attitude. I, of course, became angry. I am grateful now to that person who did. I would still be immersing myself in this negative energy if I didn't become aware of it.

The following reflections are about what shame, guilt and self-hatred did to my life.

Shame, guilt, and self-hatred

The most beautiful thing about my spirit and the Light is that they define who I am. Shame, guilt and self-hatred are imposters telling me lies about who I am. They highjack my voice and speak to me in the "I" pronoun stealing my right and the right of the Light to define my identity. They force me to believe lies about myself. They trick me into shaming myself with manipulations and lies and into everything they can to make me feel guilty about who I am. And they are able to do this because I allow fear to dwell in the seed of my identity.

Out of the three, the most damaging is self-hatred because it speaks to me as if it were me. It disguises itself behind my voice. It judges me, beats me up, makes me desire to be someone different, and takes the truth to manipulate me, to shame me and to make me feel guilty. You do not believe me? Every time we say to ourselves: "I'm a loser," or "I'm not smart enough," or

"I'm not good enough," or "I'm too ugly," or "I'm too fat," or "I'm too old," or "I've got the wrong skin color," or "I don't have class," or "nobody will like my art/music," or "I'm not worth it" or "I will never accomplish my dreams," or "nobody will listen to me," or any other judgement like this, its purpose is to shame you, hate you and make you feel guilty. This type of negative energy will quickly destroy your self-esteem, your dreams, and your strength.

Stealing, killing, and destroying "my" identity is the number one goal of self-hatred. It will use anybody including myself, to beat me up to a pulp until I doubt who I am and where I am going. It confuses me about my abilities, my skills and my dreams. It makes me feel like a loser and will make me repeat it in my mind and make me feel like a failure. And even though I beg for a glimpse of mercy in my mind to make it stop when the judgement comes, the compassion never shows up because it isn't in its nature to give it to me.

A good example of how self-hatred forced itself in my life was after my divorce. This was the perfect opportunity to get me under its control because I had lost my way. I felt like a failure because I couldn't be the perfect wife. It didn't matter that my logic was telling me that my relationship could not work with an alcoholic. Somehow the expectation of myself to make it work at whatever cost was the self-flagellation that the self-hatred was pushing me to believe. It was shaming me for my failure, and I thought it was only right to punish myself for my missteps. I thought this was my voice of reasoning and unfortunately, I fell into the trap.

In my experience as a chaplain, I have seen wonderful and deserving people not accepting the gift of healing because they feel it is right to be punished for the wrongs that they have committed. This is a lie that at one point or another, we all believe. Some of us make amends to feel worthy of the freedom from guilt. Some others are still waiting for a sign to know what to do. If you are one of them, I hope you continue reading because there is hope and you do not have to believe that you are destined to be in pain.

Self-hatred is not my friend, my voice, or my identity. I am glad to know this now. Understanding that I was depleting the energy in me by allowing a virus program to speak as it were me, was the awareness I needed to get rid of the virus. Killing myself for a lie was not an option. This gave me the strength to fight back.

Shame, guilt, and self-hatred are all based on fear. When I choose fear as my source of energy to recharge my spirit, soul, and body, I am choosing negative energy. It may give me comfort or strength or assurance for a short period of time, but at the end, it is always detrimental. It leaves me confused, angry, in fear, empty and hopeless.

Chapter 6 will address a few more behaviors of negative energy.

C.O. Aguirre

Chapter 3

C.O. Aguirre

What Is Positive Energy?

W hen I started my healing journey, I realized that getting healthy would be a full-time job for a while. But I also liked this idea because I wanted to discover who I really was through the eyes of my health. I thought that a new beginning really meant re-inventing myself.

My journey started with the help of people from a few different faiths, who taught me the principles of connecting with my soul and spirit. I am most grateful to them because they showed me how to look inside of myself and apply most of the spiritual principles mentioned in this chapter. Thanks to these principles I came back to life.

In my healing journey I have learned that the most important element in my being is the spiritual component because my life energy comes from it. It gets me re-charged. It feeds me. It surrounds me with the confidence I need. When positive energy flows through me, I feel complete, at peace, hopeful, loved, and content because I know I am one with the Light.

I know this is true because since I learned to meditate and pray, and practice them every day, I received peace and hope, and I am able to fuel my healing path. If you doubt what I am saying. I'd like you to take three deep breaths and invite peace into your life. The first thing you will notice is that the thoughts in your mind will quiet. Confusion and doubt will leave, and you feel confident to tackle the day. This is what fueling my body, soul and spirit with positive energy looks like.

Recharging yourself with positive energy during your recovery from illness and or injury will make it easier for your body, soul and spirit to heal themselves. When your spirit is fed with positive energy, it's easier for the body and mind to have a positive attitude. This is what life in abundance is all about. Abundance means having a hopeful and loving attitude towards my life. This positive view will keep you healthy, invigorated, and motivated throughout any situation you face in life. This positive outlook in life can only come when you infuse yourself with positive energy.

Spiritual principles of positive energy

The following are the most important spiritual principles I have discovered, learned about and practiced in my healing journey:

Gratitude

I call gratitude a miracle maker. My attitude towards life and people used to be negative for the most part and I didn't know how to change that. It wasn't until I forced myself to write 4 reasons why I was grateful for each day that I realized how negative my attitude was. I only saw fault with everything and everyone. I never had time to see the sunrise, the sunset, the amazing work of engineering I lived in, called my body. I didn't see my faithful friends and talents. I just waited for things to happen for me.

Expecting things from people and from life was a very painful process because it always made me feel left out, abandoned and disconnected. These negative feelings became a heavy load that made me see the world as an unbearable place to live. I always wanted to be isolated because I didn't want to feel the heavy load on my shoulders.

Being grateful allowed me to see life from a different perspective. I started to see all the good things I had going for me. I actually discovered that I had a charming personality when I wasn't expecting things from people. I also noticed that I had a relentless drive to get things done and finish projects. I realized I had many gifts: creativity, problem solving skills, and motivating people just to mention a few. Little by little the way

43

I saw the world and myself changed. I wasn't someone who needed help to live my life. I was that person who could be helping others to get things done.

My days didn't pass by without me noticing the beautiful sunrises, live paintings that were done for my enjoyment. I started to see the kindness in people, not as I expected but in different ways that touch my heart because they were unexpected. Even when I broke my foot in two places, I learned to be grateful and saw the miracle that my bones healed without needing surgery. That was for sure a miracle as my orthopedist declared. Little by little, my negative attitude started to change when I started practicing gratitude every day rigorously and thanked The Light for every single thing that happened in my life. I was no longer an afterthought. I didn't feel abandoned or disconnected. People wanted to connect with me and include me in their plans. And even if they didn't include me, I didn't feel left out anymore.

I went from being a loner to grateful for being around people. I didn't feel like I had to force myself to be nice. I was grateful to be of service. I didn't have to walk around with a list of expectations to be fulfilled.

Gratitude really changed my point of view of whom I am. This in turn became a miracle maker because I started to see all the good things around me, including every single blessing that I received.

And whenever I forget being grateful, I can see me going back to that place where I feel a heavy load on my shoulders.

I do not want to go back to that place where I have to feel like a beggar. I was not born to be a poor soul. I know this because all I have to do is look at the sky and nature and realize all the mountains, the seas, the trees and flowers that I see are for my enjoyment. If nature can flourish that way, so can I if I have the right positive energy within me.

Gratitude is the gas pumping out of that positive energy that I need to be a thriving living thing. Have you ever seen a blooming flower that manages to grow between paving stones? I cannot imagine the effort that this lonely flower used to bloom but when you see it, you are surprised about the unusual "miracle." The effort and perseverance it must have taken to get to that point is to be admired. That is why it's a miracle. I want to be like that flower. No matter what the circumstances, I want to be grateful that I was full of the right energy that allows me to grow and prosper under any circumstances. And you can have that too when you have a thankful heart.

This is the power of gratitude, it made me a living miracle where I can see how the positive energy thrives within me every day. The miracle is me changing to see life from a different perspective. It's like gratitude open my eyes to see that I will always find an answer to the issues I encounter. It may not be the solution that I want, but it is the solution that will fit my circumstances. The fact that I see my life as an opportunity to be grateful, malleable and willing to see a different perspective makes me a winner, no matter what punches life throws at me. This is a miracle I do not take lightly. It's a miracle I am forever grateful to have discovered. And this miracle can be yours, too.

And to back up my experience, scientific studies say that the benefits of gratitude include: improving physical and mental health, decreasing aggression, and improving self-esteem among other benefits.

Acceptance

I used to think that acceptance was something that losers did because they had no choice. I fought practicing acceptance in my life for a long time because I thought it would bring shame into my life. The thought of adding more shame about who I was, made me cringe and I thought it would be insufferable. It wasn't enough to feel like I never had any advantage in life, I had to admit defeat in life, and everyone was going to see it. Why did I have to be humiliated even more? Would that really make me feel better? I did not think so. In my mind, I was convinced that this spiritual principle was created to brainwash people and make them slaves. I wanted nothing to do with acceptance.

It was a "coincidence" realizing what acceptance really meant. This spiritual principle was meant to give me peace and release me of the chaos and confusion I was creating in my mind. One day while I was visiting with my friend and we were baking cookies, I noticed the tender moments she had with one of her girls. I looked at them with such sadness and sorrow in my soul because I wished I had at least one tender moment like that with my mother. I do not think I ever did, or at least I do not remember.

Seeing myself in a flash that I was sinking in the sorrow, I quickly prayed under my breath: "Dear Light, I thank you that I did not experience this kind of tenderness as a child. Perhaps I did and I cannot recall. But if I never did, I thank you for it. I do not understand the reason why I couldn't, but I am quite certain that I have not gone through life not experiencing love. Not having that experience has not change at all who I am or what I am supposed to be in life. I thank you that with or without that experience I am still true to whom I am and for that I am grateful."

As soon as I finished saying those words, I realized peace entered my heart. Gratitude had brought me the miracle of acceptance. It was OK that my parents were not like those I saw on TV. I was complete and equipped to run my life today and I did not need those moments that I thought I did. It was OK to let go of that grudge that would make me blame my parents for what I thought was a lack in my life. Because after all, I wasn't lacking anything today. At that very moment I said: "Oh, so you are 'Acceptance.' Welcome to my life."

Acceptance was that surrender of letting go of the past. Those grievances that I thought I needed to validate me because I couldn't see one of them making me richer, wiser, healthier or more popular in life. They were just thoughts, things I thought would make me happy in life, but they didn't.

What I wanted deep inside was to be a special, lovable girl. I thought I needed to do or be many things to become that girl. One of them was to find the perfect little black dress. This perfect black dress would help me find prince charming and make me the happiest girl ever. This was the fantasy running through my head when I met my first boyfriend. He was a simple man who just wanted to make me happy. But the fantasy in my head was that prince charming taking me out to incredible places and me wearing that little black dress. I remember when my first boyfriend took me out to dinner. He didn't have a lot of money, so we ended up going to a small restaurant. This was not exactly my fantasy and during the entire dinner, all I could think of was that I wasn't having that dinner I imagined in my fantasy. I completely missed seeing the way he looked at me, that look that sparkled and infused me with life. That was what I needed to feel happy at that moment. But I discarded it for a little fantasy that dared me to fit in that dress and find a sophisticated man who would show me the world.

When I finally found that little black dress and fit in it, I went out with many boys, many of them European and well educated. I ended up marrying the most extraordinary, intelligent European man just to find out I had missed the mark. I wanted my marriage to work but no matter what I did, it didn't last because he was an alcoholic with a lot of rage inside. I had ignored all the red flags and built my relationship on a fantasy.

Funny to think about it now when I realize that I didn't need that little black dress to find someone to love me. What I needed was to "accept" me and that I was lovable no matter what I was wearing. I did not need a fantasy to find love or for someone to fall in love with me. Coming to terms with letting the fantasy go was acceptance.

When I finally let the black dress fantasy go, it did not bring me shame, nor pain, nor affliction. I just knew that the fantasy was something that would not work for me. Knowing this liberated me from being someone I wasn't meant to be. I became free to express my creativity and explore whom I really was. Acceptance of the real me has allowed me to travel to places I never imagined I could visit.

Acceptance became the realization that all things that had happened to me in the past, good or bad, were that motivation to find the Light within me because I knew there was more to life than just aching and confusion and the feeling of emptiness inside.

Acceptance became the connection with the Light, that feeling when you surrender because you know you do not have the answers and you "renounce" the right to find out all the answers because it is impossible.

Acceptance became the conviction that I do not need to know all the answers and I do not have to be right all the time. Acceptance gave me the craving for peace because that is the only thing my soul and spirit wanted to have in the first place.

Acceptance became the answer to all my problems because no problem, no worry, no doubt, no fear, no feeling is worth letting go of the peace that soothes my body, mind and spirit.

Acceptance is letting go of the past, of the things I think I should have had or been. Acceptance helps me let go of the expectations of the future and clears the path to new beginnings.

Acceptance gets activated by gratitude and between the two of them, they open my eyes to see the richness of my day – the sunrise, the sunset, a kind smile, and the joy of being alive.

Still not sure if acceptance works? Scientific studies show that acceptance supports physical and mental health, brings inner peace, improves problem solving abilities and contributes to healthier relationships.

Willingness

This is a word that implies commitment. I do not think there is a person on earth who has ran away from commitment like I have. After my first marriage fell apart, I did not want to make the same mistakes again. I saw all the red flags and still went ahead and made a commitment to give my life completely to someone who had no desire to be a grownup. I cried bitter tears after I saw my mistakes and sworn never to let another man hurt me again. I thought I was doing the right thing by protecting myself and to a certain extent, I was. But when I locked my heart and threw away the key, I also blocked my soul from receiving love and affection from anyone around me.

For a long time, I walked around with a soul and spirit who were starved, and I just ignored the signs because I was too afraid to commit to trust again. You see, love is the positive energy that breathes life into our soul and spirit like oxygen does with the body. This is why we crave for relationships. So, when I famished my soul and spirit, I allowed the negative energy to feed them. Sure, it felt good for a while to be in control and not let anybody hurt me but what I did not see was what that negative energy was doing to me. I started to become mistrusting, suspicious, irritated and distant among other things. That wall I built trapped me inside and my spirit couldn't connect with the spirit of life anymore. All of a sudden, I started to feel like my life had no meaning.

At the time, I was going to a religious group. For a while I felt useful because I was told I needed to volunteer doing this or that to show my commitment. Volunteering helped me reconnect with people, but it was only a temporary fix. My soul and my spirit still felt empty and lonely.

I didn't know what the answer was back then, but I clearly understood that I wasn't finding what I needed. I wished I could trust someone to open up my heart so the Light would come in. It took me a few years of literally going in full chaos in my head to finally find a spiritual group of women who honestly practiced the spiritual principles of the Light. They were kind to me, they did not judge me, not even once. They let me grow at my own pace and encouraged me to find the truth within me. It was one of the hardest things I did, but I let go of the walls.

I became vulnerable, I cried a lot, and for the first time I understood my spirit was poor and fragile. These women earned my trust, my love and my commitment by validating that fragile person they saw. I started a personal journal and wrote about the spiritual principles I was learning about in the group. Little by little I saw how gratitude became a miracle maker in my life. Acceptance became the answer to all my problems and kindness was the antidote to anger. I noticed how my attitude was so different when I purposely meditated and prayed every day.

It became clear to me that if I were to make a commitment, my spiritual health was the one I should choose. A commitment to see myself centered, well and at peace. That became the promise that would steer me to make the right decisions in my life. A pledge that was worth my time, my effort, and my dedication.

But knowing me, I just knew that I would forget my promise if I didn't have a spiritual program in place. A program that included daily prayer and meditation and the willingness to commit and be responsible for myself every day. For some reason, my soul does not like commitments. I am a free spirit. And as much as I love that part of me, I know now that without the influx of positive energy every day, I go back to that dark place where I am disconnected, lonely and confused. So, the choice was between having peace or chaos. A commitment became reasonable when I saw what was at stake.

Establishing and cementing the willingness to practice the spiritual principles is a must in order to be successful. Making that commitment to be "willing" to take care of myself is called "love for self." Not making the commitment for "willingness" is like cutting all ties with the real me, with the person I am meant to be. It's like wanting to live in the darkness where the truth is not spoken, and I do not see myself anymore.

It is a good thing to commit to me because I deserve it. We all deserve to be taken care of, to be respected, to be looked after and that behavior starts with us by making a commitment to ourselves to be willing to do it.

Willingness is the key that opens the door for loving ourselves. Even if you think you do not deserve it, still make the commitment. You will see love blooming out of you.

Still not sure if willingness is for you? Scientific studies show that willingness is the key to successfully learn how to change behavior.

Love

This is a word that I did not understand. I say this because when I think of love, the first image that comes to mind is a couple being in love or intimate. The levels of love go beyond that passionate love. And love is more than the love of a parent for their children.

In order to understand what I am saying I want to tell you this story. I have a friend who is a therapist. We are very close. She became my person to go to when I decided to start putting the right food into my body. She would give me advice on eating properly because I have the tendency to be an emotional eater. At that time, I was having a lot of "emotional" moments at work and my consumption of sugar became evident in my weight. We were driving to go out to dinner one day and she said to me, "I see that you are gaining weight. The day you learn to love yourself is the day you will not have the need to overeat." I wasn't sure what she meant. Love myself? I was just trying to distract myself from the drama at work. I had the right to indulge a little because I worked hard. Why would she tell me I did not love myself? I did not understand this concept until two more years passed and I learned about self-hatred.

I was very judgmental of myself and didn't even know about it. I would put unattainable expectations on myself and was constantly doubting myself. I was afraid of people not liking me and the list went on and on about the negative image I had of myself. I thought it was a well-kept secret but to my dismay, people knew about it, just like my friend who told me I needed to love myself.

Love for self

I have discovered in the last few years that loving me is the most important person I can love and if I only had the capacity to love one person on this earth it should be me. No romantic love, no parental love, no best-friend love can compare or even come close to what it means to love me.

This amazing beautiful love that I have for myself manifest not in a narcissistic way but exactly the opposite. In this love, I respect my body, soul and spirit. I make sure I feed me in a healthy way. I also maintain my body, soul and spirt and do whatever it takes for me to be at peace. I also invite hope and love into my life, especially at those moments when I feel stressed and tired.

I purposely and audibly express love for myself. What does that look like? I try not criticizing myself but encouraging me for doing the best I could have done. I express gratitude for whom I am and do not wish I would be someone else. This love is a quest to find out who I am, what I am capable of, what I can give to this world and be the best person I can be. This love nurtures myself and gives myself the opportunity to make mistakes without judging me, criticizing me or thinking that I am less than. I love myself by not being a perfectionist but by praising the work I have done no matter what the end result. Doing this will be the best example you can give your kids.

I am grateful for the person I am today and for all the mistakes that I have made in the past and I do not look back because I am the best outcome of myself for going through the issues and situations from the past. I accept the person I am today, and I bless me for being this amazing work of art and engineering. I am grateful that I am unique in every single way.

I am kind to myself by getting rid of negative energy in my body, soul or spirit because I know being filled with positive energy is what I need to find my way in life.

Loving myself with passion is understanding that this love will automatically transfer to all people I encounter. They deserve my respect and kindness. And I understand that being at peace and harmony with them is not for their benefit but for mine.

Just as I practice no judgement with myself, I stop judging the world, not for their benefit but for mine. I understand that judging myself and the world only brings me suffering, disappointment, pain and isolation. My job is not to fix others or to control others. My job is to bring peace and hope into my life, and I achieve this by bringing peace and hope into the relationships I develop. I understand that I must be kind to myself and the world to avoid falling into the black hole of negative energy.

This is what love is all about – understanding that I must take care of me so that this love will ripple to the rest of the people, the world and the universe. This love manifests in the kindness I show to the people around me. Peace, hope and love start with me and that is one of my contributions to the universe – to have a peaceful and loving planet.

Loving me means loving everyone that I come in contact with – this is why it is the most amazing love! I end up touching my partner, kids, family, neighbors, my community, my country, and the world when I love myself.

Love for the Light

This love is also very important because when I love myself, I am also loving the Light. When I love myself, I am in agreement with the light that I am "perfect," without being a perfectionist. When I love the Light, I accept that I am unique and special because that is the way the Light made me. When I love myself, I understand that the Light made this amazing person that I call me. When I love myself, I understand that the Light created a beautiful being equipped with everything I need to discover who I am without judging the reflection that I see on the mirror.

Loving the Light for the most part for me is an act of wonder that I am a very small part of the universe and still I am one of the most amazing complex beings that we know of. Loving that energy that gives me life and equips me to experience life is to stand in awe when I realize I am an extension of the Light. The only way I can express my love to the Light is with gratitude for all the amazing daily things that I sometimes take for granted.

Loving the Light is understanding that when I do not love myself, I do not love the Light either or anything connected with the Light. Loving the Light makes me aware that having this attitude of disdain against myself and everything connected with the Light, separates me from the Light and this is an attitude I must avoid at all costs.

And just as I love myself with passionate love, I also love the Light for allowing me to discover the true love inside of me. For showing me the way to kindness and hope because without them I would not know who I am.

The Light is the essence of love and discovering what this means is an adventure I do not want to miss.

I love the Light for giving me the miracle of "being grateful" because by practicing gratitude, I discover my life is full of miracles, surprises, and blessings.

I love the Light because each day I wake up is a reminder of the beautiful gift of life. I see the sunrise and I realize the skies were painted for my pleasure, to start my day with hope and to remind me that my day will be filled with color and beauty.

I love the Light for giving me senses to experience life through aromas, sight, tastes, touch, and hearing. Being able to do this has made my life rich.

I love the Light because I have found people who want to be close to me and like me even though sometimes, I didn't like myself and didn't think I belonged.

I love the Light for not giving up on me and waiting until I was ready to hear the truth that I must fill my life with positive energy in order to feel the love of the Light.

In a few words, love for the Light is a self-discovery of whom I am and the world around me. It's accepting myself and the people around me. It's respecting myself and the people around me. It's being kind to myself and understanding that I belong. It's extending the same kindness to the people around me. Understanding that this world was made for my pleasure and I express my love back to the Light by respecting it just like I respect myself.

Still not sure if love can give you a better life? Scientific studies show that love improves physical and mental health, reduces depression, anxiety, and substance abuse, lowers levels of physical pain, promotes faster healing, fosters a happier life, lowers stress levels and gives the immune system a boost.

Kindness

For a long time, I confused pleasing people with kindness and I never wanted to be kind because I thought it was a sign of weakness and everyone would just step on me and take advantage of me. I am happy to say that this belief has been rectified. Kindness is not the same as being an enabler. Kindness has to do with respect and it always starts with me first.

What do I mean by kindness starts with me? True kindness starts with me because I must assess the boundaries of respect for myself when I make decisions about me and others. It may not feel nice saying no to me when I want a new pair of shoes that are out of my budget but out of respect for me and my needs, I must say no to indulgence. The same with a friend or relative who keeps asking me to help them financially when my budget cannot afford it. I must ask the question and be honest. Why do I want to help when I know I cannot do it? Is it because I am afraid that they will gossip about me not being a nice person? Is it that I am afraid that they will not like me? Is it that I want something in return and not just help out of the kindness of my heart? Out of respect for me, I have to see my needs first and then see if there is another way I can help.

This reminds me about how the flight attendants give you instructions before a plane takes off. If the cabin goes low on pressure, the oxygen masks are released. They tell you to put the oxygen mask on first and then help your child or the person next to you put theirs on. Kindness is the same. I have to make sure I am in good condition and safe to help others. If I must say "no" when someone asks me for help or I see someone in need and I cannot help, it's not that I do not feel their pain and need. When I cannot help someone, I still can find someone who can help them or pray for the Light to send someone to help.

If I help because I feel like I need to please them, then I need to rethink my concept of kindness to myself. Otherwise, I will end up being resentful and that is not kindness to anybody, especially to myself because resentment is not a good energy to store in my body.

Kindness has to do with empathy for myself first. And what is empathy? The way I understand it is to have compassion about the situation that a person is going through and share in the feelings of it and if I have the desire to help them, I must understand my needs first so I can be of service to them. Using the oxygen mask example, I must have my oxygen mask on first before I can help anyone else. Otherwise, I am not help to myself or others.

A few weeks ago, I was journaling in my healing diary, and I was asking to understand what kindness to myself meant and the answer came almost instantly: "Kindness is the antidote to anger." I started to chew on this in all my meditations because I didn't understand what it meant. One morning, during my meditation, I felt encouraged to seek within me to look for anger. When my meditation was over, I thought about this and I kept thinking, "I do not have any anger issues." The thought of me being angry was preposterous. I was not angry. Later that day when I was driving coming back from work, this person cut in front of me in a very erratic way. This energy of anger rose in my gut and I wanted to show this person how dangerous they were. I started to follow them trying to catch up to them and all of a sudden a voice in my head said: "What are you doing? Is your health and safety worth throwing away just to show this person how wrong they are and how right you are? What kind of anger is this?" To my dismay, I knew the answers and they were not pretty. At that moment I had to choose kindness to myself and to the other driver and let go of my desire to get "justice" because accumulating that kind of energy is the kind of energy that makes me sick, confused, lonely and overall blinds me from the important things in life. Does the other driver need the kindness of me letting go of their infraction? If I see it from the justice point of view, of course not. But kindness stated with me putting the mask of oxygen on and make myself safe, it was not something I could ignore. I could see that the other driver needed help because driving erratically like that is not the behavior of a person who has peace and hope in their mind. So, I chose kindness, blessed the driver and I let go of my right to claim justice. I did this for my safety first and then because I could understand that the other driver needed someone to be kind to them.

Now, I do the same when people push my buttons. I put the oxygen mask of positive energy on and bless people. If I feel that my boundaries are trespassed, I take the following steps:

-       I assess the situation really quickly to see if anything was destroyed, damaged or stolen from me.

-       I say a quick prayer for my peace of mind to be covered (see prayer for peace at the end of the book for a quick reference).

`   In kindness, I vocalized that my boundaries have been trespassed and ask for the other person(s) to respect my boundaries and return what was taken from me.

-       I let go of my expectation that I will get justice because that expectation only makes me get angry if things do not go the way I want.

- The Light always brings balance and prosperity when I practice positive energy, so I wrap my mind in this spiritual principle to keep my peace of mind and do not allow fear to convince me that my loses are great and I need to fight back.

- I show kindness to people throughout the process of resolving the issue, keeping my peace of mind and hope as the priority.

You might be thinking that this strategy of solving problems is weak and flawed. Of course, there are some people who do not care about taking somebody else's property or damaging it. They may even vocalize that you are weak and will not respect you. You may think that they are getting away with it, but before you label kindness as weak, consider two things:

1.   You cannot control anybody but yourself.

2.   If you allow fear and doubt to control your mind, you will lose more than the property that was damaged or stolen from you. You will lose your mental health, your physical health and anger and fear will take over you. Is some possession worth losing your health and life over it?

Kindness is not letting people walk all over me when I decide to show mercy. Kindness is the strength to let go of the "right I have" when I'm injured by others, not out of fear, but out of love for myself because my wellbeing is more important than any other alternative.

Exercising kindness is not letting people steal from me, control me, or stepping all over me. Kindness is understanding that people may be in pain or injured, which is why they are trespassing my boundaries. And after I have gotten rid of the anger and let go of the "right" to get justice, I decide to deal with the situation with a cool head and a kind heart.

The miracle of kindness is not that you let go of the right to get justice. The miracle is that you let go of the anger because you understand that rage makes you ill and destroys your mental health. The miracle is that you see the whole picture and chose life for your sake and the sake of the trespassers. The miracle is that you choose to love the trespassers above your need to be right. Therefore, the miracle of kindness is that you chose to love your neighbor as you love yourself. Practicing this spiritual principle will bring back into your life what was stolen from you and much more.

Hard to believe that kindness can improve your life? Scientific studies show that kindness prevents inflammation of the body associated with cancer, diabetes, pain, obesity, and migraines. Studies have also shown that kindness reduces stress, anxiety, blood pressure and improves mental health.

Forgiveness

Having the ability to forgive is a miracle in my book. I do not think any human being has the capacity to forgive. And it's not like we do not want to. We just do not have the gene for it. Forgiveness is a gift from the Light because it doesn't come naturally to us. We need a special programming in our mind to be able to do it.

What is forgiveness? I have heard many definitions of forgiveness in religious arenas, my counselor sessions and support groups. The following definition is a collection of thoughts from all these places. Forgiveness is releasing my feelings of resentment and vengeance against those who harmed me without considering whether they deserve it or not.

When I started my healing journey, I had a very hard time with this definition. Why would I let people off the hook? It wasn't fair. I suffered domestic abuse in the relationship with my ex-husband. He never hit me, but the verbal abuse was so great, that for months after we separated, I got paralyzed when I heard a man raising his voice to a woman. What would forgiving him look like? Would that mean that I had to accept him back into my life and put up with his abuse? Would it mean to forget all he made me go through only to fall victim to someone else and experience it once again? Forgiveness certainly didn't make sense to me besides being unfair.

I had the same questions about forgiveness when I became the victim of sexual harassment at the workplace. I put up with the sexual insinuations because I needed the job. But being passive and letting it go for so long did not help at all. I felt trapped and manipulated and with reason because sexual harassment is not about sex but control. I became afraid and angry about this person's manipulation. I had so much anger against this person, who not only wouldn't take no for an answer but who also blocked me from getting another job inside the company as well as outside the company. He was getting away with destroying my life, doing something that was punishable by law and nobody was holding him accountable for his wrongdoings. It wasn't like I was the only woman he pursued at work. In fact, I think I was the only woman who did not sleep with him. But no one else was punished but me for not giving in.

The anger that I felt was not just against this person. I was angry beyond belief that the company knew about the sexual activity of this man and the favors given to the women sleeping with him. He was promoting these women and the company did nothing to stop it. But when it came to me requesting to move to another department, the answer was always no. And when I hinted about the sexual harassment, they let me go. Why did I have to release the company and this man from all legal accountability? And why was my spiritual mentor suggesting that I had to ask forgiveness from him for keeping resentment against him? Forgiveness certainly did not look like something I even wanted to consider.

We do not have in us the ability to exercise forgiveness. Our mind or soul is wired to "fix and execute computer code" so when I feel that someone trespass my boundaries, injures me or wrongs me, the code in my head says to "fix it and execute" which translates into "stop that person and/or get even." There are many ways to get even. One is to get angry and respond in an aggressive manner. Another way is to plan for revenge and wait for the right moment to get even. Another way is to hold resentment and not do anything to the other person, but the resentment boils down inside my guts in hopes that something bad will happen to the other person but the only one who ends up sick is me for holding negative energy inside of me.

I think just like me, I have met a lot of people in my healing journey that struggled with forgiveness. Until one day, in a support group, I heard this person discuss how their life was changing for the better all because they entertained the idea of forgiveness. They felt "free." I know I had heard the word "free" before but somehow, I did not believe freedom would come from forgiveness. But I had seen this person struggle with forgiveness just like me and there they were…something inside of them changed. That's when I opened my heart to the possibility of forgiving.

I must say that I entered into the "possibility" of forgiving in a very cautious way. I asked my counselor a lot of questions about what exactly I had to give up to forgive. I asked this question to my friends as well and in support groups and started to read about it. I wanted to know for sure what I was getting in return from dropping my claim of getting justice. I thought it was a perfectly normal, responsible, "adult way" to go about it. Some of them had answers and others did not or the answers I got were not to my liking. The best definition I came across was from the online magazine Greater Good Science Center at UC Berkeley (greatergood.berkeley.edu). This is what captured my eye:

"Forgiveness brings the forgiver peace of mind and frees him or her from corrosive anger… it empowers you to recognize the pain you suffered without letting that pain define you, enabling you to heal and move on with your life."

I read this paragraph over and over again to try to absorb the meaning of it. I do not remember hearing this before, but I am sure at some point my counselor said this to me. But I never heard it that clearly. I guess my heart was not open then so I could not comprehend the meaning of the freedom being offered to me. This forgiving business was not about forcing me to do something that I did not want to do. It was about validating my pain and the offense perpetrated against me and then me being able to move on.

I understand now that forgiveness is a higher choice that my brain was not able to get because of two reasons. The first one is that when my boundaries are trespassed, my natural response is anger. If I choose to keep the anger because I want revenge of some form, the anger is immediately fed with negative energy and the resentment most likely will never leave me. The second reason is because forgiveness is a positive spiritual principle. Unless I actively ask for it and practice it, forgiveness doesn't come my way.

Forgiveness brings more than just itself. Allowing forgiveness in my life gives me peace of mind, love, and respect for myself. This stops the voice of fear telling me that if I do not embrace "justice," people will continue to injure me. Forgiveness gives me the strength to disengage from people who are toxic and not safe for me so I won't be injured anymore. Forgiveness gives me the strength to protect my identity, so I won't give the injurer the right to define myself. Knowing all these things, I am able to let go of the offenses and not accumulate negative energy inside my body.

Forgiveness makes me understand that the Light and I are the only ones who have the right to define who I am, not the people who have injured me or the injuries that I have endured. It is very empowering to understand this because freedom and power are released when I allow forgiveness into my life.

After I understood all these things, I decided to forgive my ex-husband, my former manager, and my former place of work. I also forgave myself for keeping resentment, such negative energy inside of me. I can say with certainty that I am truly free from the resentment I had against my ex-husband because our paths have crossed since then, and it doesn't bother me any longer the insults he still spits out when he is drunk. To my surprise, I do not entertain his words anymore because I know they do not define me. Once in a while I pray for him, that he will find peace just as I have. Choosing forgiveness is a very personal choice and I hope someday my ex-husband finds the inspiration and strength to make that choice for himself.

Does forgiveness mean to release people from legal accountability? I think this is a personal choice that needs to be taken with advice from a spiritual mentor and therapist. One has to think it over and weigh the pros and cons and then decide what is best for them. As for me, I decided not to pursue legal action against my former place of work or my former manager regarding the sexual harassment issue. I decided that my peace of mind was more important than having to drag myself into a courtroom for years and having people question my integrity. I pray that they will find peace and start protecting the people who work under them rather than doing the opposite.

If you feel legal action is necessary, do take action. Seek advice not only from lawyers but also from a spiritual counselor and a therapist and anyone else who may be able to give you a better perspective on how to go about with the lawsuit. Still, make sure your heart does not hold any resentment. Make sure you do not hold any negative energy in your body, soul, or spirit. Your health is the most important thing so, protect yourself from any negative energy throughout the legal process.

What a journey it was to learn the meaning of forgiveness. It is a powerful spiritual principle that sets us free from letting the pain of injustice define us. This spiritual principle is a gift that describes the true nature of the Light. It takes humility and surrender of the ego to receive it. And even though it may feel too much to give up, the healing we receive is the most extraordinary gift because it not only heals the body but also restores the soul and spirit.

Still have a hard time believing that forgiveness is a miracle and a gift from the Light? Scientific studies show that forgiveness improves mental health, lowers levels of chronic pain and chronic illness, releases anxiety, stress, and aggression, boosts the immune system, and improves heart health and self-esteem among other benefits.

Peace

This principle is one of the most awesome gifts I have received. It does not have to do with canceling the noise around me. Au contraire, it means being able to be in the middle of a storm (physically or figuratively speaking) and being able to not lose my cool. My mind is at peace, so I am able to make the right decisions and move out of the path of the storm with confidence.

Feeling protected and safe in the middle of the storm is what I define as having peace of mind. It is in that state of peace that my mind is able to hear the voice of the Light. What do I mean by this? It is when my mind is at peace that all chaos, confusion, doubt, anxiety, worry, stress, and fear are shut down and the voice of confidence, trust, courage, and kindness guide my path.

Science studies show that peace of mind makes a person happier, protects the mind from aging, improves mental health, and lowers the levels of inflammation making the immune system stronger.

When my mind is not at peace, I open the door for negative energy to enter my mind, spirit and body, and I take off the protection I have against disease. My house needs peace to have energy efficiency. This means that when I lose my peace, my positive energy begins to leak because I open the door to negativity.

Negative energy only comes to steal, kill, and destroy my positive energy and in turn, my being. This is exactly what fear and all emotions derived from fear do to us. They steal our happiness, our health, our peace of mind leaving us with a life we do not want to live. The best way to prevent a positive energy leakage is to buckle up our peace of mind and defend it. How do I do this? By immersing myself into positive energy and understanding that the Light and its energy are what I need to overcome any situation.

Peace will bring us safety and security, and this is what we need to make optimal decisions for our life and prevent our positive energy from leaving us.

Still think peace is not for you? Scientific studies show that inner peace or peace of mind increases intelligence, decreases the aging process, slows down age-related mental decline, enhances memory and concentration, improves digestion, elevates the levels of happiness, and boosts the immune system.

Hope

This principle is also a gift. It is a feeling of trust and optimism that the right answers will come. I took hope for granted most of my life because I didn't realize that it came attached to another gift I had, creative problem solving. You see, hope usually comes in the form of having an idea about finding a solution to the problem we have. If we need a job, hope comes in the form of finding job leads and ways to help us get a job. Sometimes hope comes when we find a creative way to solve the problem. A creative way to get that job we want would be sending a video with our resume highlighting the reasons why we are the best candidate for the job. These ideas and creative ways to get us out of a tight spot are like getting a shot of hope.

I always thought these bursts of creativity were something that everyone had. I didn't realize this was not the case until I noticed at work that my ideas would always end up being credited to someone else. I started to lose confidence in myself and think that these bursts of creativity that helped others were just a waste of time.

Once I stopped doing what brought me hope, contentment and fulfillment, my life started to feel empty. I had stopped the one flow of positive energy in my life that made me look forward to the future with optimism. I thought that by giving away the golden eggs, I had killed Mother Goose. What I didn't know was that the Light was an endless source of creativity. And all I had to do was to refill my spirit and soul with new creativity, and new hope would come. Creativity and hope were given to me to help me but also to help others, so it was okay to give the golden eggs away. In time, hope made the golden eggs fall into the right hands and the future I hoped for came to pass.

Some scientific studies say that hope releases endorphins in the brain getting rid of pain and producing happiness. Science has also discovered that hope generates resilience and opens the door for self-healing. Science may not know where hope comes from, but I can tell you that trusting the Light has everything to do with it. When my human spirit receives hope, good things come my way no matter where I am and what I am going through because I'm filling up my tank with positive energy.

Hope is the vision of all the possible good things that can come to my life and that includes my goals and dreams. Hope also refers to envisioning a positive outcome when I am going through a challenging circumstance. Hope acts like a protector when I feel vulnerable and out of control. It becomes my strength when I need to run the extra-mile and I don't feel like I can make it. Hope is a healer when I feel my body is giving up. Hope is a friend when I feel nobody wants to be around me. Hope is a companion that will cheer me up and whisper in my ear the good news that wait for me when I cross the finish line.

I do not think I can live without hope now that I know its benefits are endless. There will be stormy days ahead and I want to be prepared and have a storehouse full of hope that I can embrace when I need to trust and be optimistic about the future.

Not sure about hope yet? According to scientific studies, hope lowers the levels of anxiety, depression, and stress, relieves joint pain, improves physical and mental health, boosts the immune system, and improves self-esteem.

Self-control

Self-control is not an emotion but the ability to control emotions and behaviors. Why is this a positive energy principle? Because strong negative energy like fear and anger does not ask permission to come into your mind, soul, and spirit; it just forces itself like a bully breaking all your boundaries. In order to be prepared for those moments when negative energy attacks you, you must have a strategy called "self-control."

When self-control is broken, so to speak, the brain reveals behavior like compulsions and obsessions because self-control is not fed by positive energy but by negative energy making one lose control of their emotions and behaviors. For example, when we are afraid or angry and the emotions overwhelm us, it is hard to stop eating carbohydrates.

Is this too hard to believe? Scientists say that the place in the brain where emotions and behaviors are controlled is the pre-frontal cortex. This part of the brain in people with OCD (obsessive compulsive disorder) does not respond the same as other people. The underlying emotion in compulsive and repetitive behavior is to prevent that dreaded event or situation playing in the mind. In other words, fear and stress cause the brain to freeze and not respond when self-control is required.

The good news is that there are effective spiritual programs based on positive energy that help release the mind from that freeze and the fear that has a grip on it. Support groups like 12-step groups are recommended by counselors to help control behaviors and compulsions that cause addictions. These support groups teach that addictions are fed by negative energy that can be stopped by surrendering the will to the Light and allow its positive energy to arrest the addiction one day at a time. Surrendering the will to the Light is the key to having self-control. An amazing miracle, really, if you ask me.

One of the best tools I found to strengthen my self-control was meditation. The best way it was explained to me was that during meditation we see thoughts as clouds floating around. Instead of taking every cloud I see, I just let them be and let them pass. This may seem simple, but it takes a lot of practice and trust in the Light. Being able to control your emotions is the same spiritual principle that meditation uses with thoughts. You see the emotions rise. Those fueled by negative energy pass by. You only engage with those fueled by positive energy. You surrender your right to engage with negative emotions and trust the Light that the outcome from choosing positive energy will benefit you more. Does this really work? Yes, it does. I am a living testimony that it does work.

Self-control is a principle for preventive care. We want to be able to walk out of the house each morning with confidence that we are ready to face the world. We visualize self-control and self-loving in our meditations in the morning and practice it throughout the day when we exercise positive energy.

No matter how tempting it is to get scared when hearing the news about a pandemic, for example, we must be able to stop the emotions because self-control is a behavior that says: "I love myself, so I will not let my mind be inundated with these negative thoughts."

Self-control is the strategy that allows us to choose what thoughts can capture our emotions, especially when we are taken by surprise. Self-control will give the wisdom and strength to our mind from letting go of the peace of mind needed to make the right choices in a difficult situation. Self-control is like a weapon that weakens the power of fear and anger and any negative energy trying to seize our mind and emotions. Self-control is the best defense we can carry around to protect ourselves and the people around us. It will give us in return respect and self-esteem.

Still not sure about self-control? According to studies, self-control improves mental health focus and decision making, makes you live longer, reduces impulsive behavior, improves physical and mental health, and increases resilience.

Recycling

This principle is behavior in nature. We see it all over the earth. The most famous recyclers in nature are hermit crabs. They do not grow their shells. Instead, they reclaim discarded shells from other marine life to protect themselves. But they do not stop there. When they need a new home, they will use glass bottles, plastic tops, cans, or any materials they find at the bottom of the ocean that will shelter them. In their world, nothing goes to waste.

We also use this recycling principle to redirect the purpose of many man-made materials like plastic. When a plastic bag has fulfilled its purpose, it goes to recycling to begin a new way of being useful. This is the kind of recycling we will be talking about in this chapter.

There are no scientific studies about "recycling yourself." Instead, I offer the benefits found in studies of a spiritual principle close in meaning: "resilience." Scientific studies about resilience lowers levels of stress, elevates levels of happiness, improves mental health and increases self-esteem. "Recycling yourself" will bring much more than resilience. It will give you a new life.

How does recycle apply to me? Before I explain this, I want to tell you about a couple of losses in my life. After my cancer treatment, I felt incomplete, like my womanhood had been stolen and I was, "leftovers" of the person I used to be. I thought my life was over. I even called myself "damaged goods." I knew these feelings had a lot of negative energy and I did not know what to do about it. It reminded me that I had felt this once before when I was going through the loss of my marriage and my best friend. I felt like "damaged goods." Back then I felt so depressed thinking that so many parts inside of me had died along with so many dreams that it made me an incomplete person.

Then I thought, if I recovered my sense of self before, I know I can do it again. I just need to know how to do it. I started searching for the answer as if my life depended on it because it did.

A week later, I went to my support group for people recovering from cancer. My friend talked about having the same feelings, but she had something else I did not have. Her point of view shocked me to my core. She was a "recycling person" in her spare time. Wherever she went, she would find something to recycle.

Going through her recovery, my friend felt many times incomplete. But she decided to change that feeling by affirming and continuing her purpose in life by doing recycling full time. This had become not just her hobby but her purpose in life. She was good at it and she was going to focus on recycling all kinds of things with whatever time she had after taking care of her daughter.

This idea of recycling would not leave me. It never occurred to me that I could do something good with what was left of me.

My friend used the word "recycling." The meaning of the word grew stronger in my heart the more I thought about it.

Days passed by and after journaling in my diary about recycling, I discovered that putting these two words together, "recycling" and "myself" was not such a crazy idea. My soul, my spirit and body were still strong in so many ways and there was no reason to throw them away. I still had my creativity, my drive, my dreams and nothing was stopping me from doing something with them. That day I decided to find out what I was most passionate about.

I remember trying so many things. I started to do photography, writing, shooting a pilot for children's programming, and even forming a non-profit organization. I dedicated time and money to explore each option and see what made me get up every morning. I went through all and none of them took me to the highs I was expecting. But doing all of them made me complete. I continued to pursue them all and one morning I got the most unexpected answer. "Being a healer" were the words playing in my head. I had been praying for healing for others in the past 10 years of my life. These years were the most rewarding years. I witnessed people heal, recover, improve, and even expand their lives, because they found more than healing. They found peace and purpose. The Light changed their life for the better. I was stopped in my tracks and I knew I had found my purpose. That is when I decide to write about my healing journey because I knew someone may benefit from my experience.

Being recycled is a beautiful way I see myself being reborn. I have the best parts of me, and I get to use them for good. I have found a higher purpose than what I had before in my life. I know it is true for me that the Light has redesigned me to function more efficiently and with a higher purpose. Every day I fill myself up with positive energy and continue throughout the day, I never know when someone in need will cross my path and I will need to share hope with this person. As a healer, I understand that my positive energy is the best possession that the Light has given me. Sharing with those in need of healing has become a goal that fulfills every part of me. I found my purpose just like my friend did, by using what is left in me to the best of my abilities.

If you are also recovering from illness or going through it and feel incomplete, cut short of your time on earth or just unable to feel whole, I invite you to think about what is "left" of you...the essence of your being, the most precious thing your spirit can give you. What is left of us is not a waste, we were not short-changed. We have been given an opportunity to see the most beautiful version of ourselves by rechanneling the best parts of us. I invite you to open up yourself to discover that beautiful being that is willing to blossom out of you. You are a living miracle worthy of appreciation just like we admire the sunrise or the sunset.

How to receive positive energy

Positive energy is more than having a positive outlook on life, having happy thoughts and positive affirmations. Positive energy is the essence of the Light: love, gratitude, peace, hope, kindness, acceptance, inclusion, self-esteem, forgiveness, healing, serenity, happiness (not pleasure), self-control and faith.

Receiving positive energy is not about knowing about these traits. It's about practicing them. And how do I go about obtaining each of these traits? Do I pray for them, do I wish for them? Do I study them? The mission of this book is to teach you how to bring positive energy into your life by developing a connection with the Light and practicing the positive energy principles.

The following chapters talk about all the places where one can fill their tank with positive energy. But most important how to make that connection with the Light because without it, it will be hard to receive the positive energy that comes your way every day. This connection sometimes comes from unexpected places like other people. Yes, people. These encounters may be pleasant, unpleasant or just annoying. But that desire to connect with the Light will propel you to want to get out of your comfort zone. This will make you stronger and build your trust in the Light.

Being around people will also remind you of things you must do. For example, when you are depleted of positive energy for a very long time, sometimes you cannot recognize what kindness for yourself looks like. Being around people who practice these spiritual principles will encourage you to pursue them as well. It will also teach you to divide your "positive energy to-do list" into small bites.

The following is the list of activities that will open up your spirit to receive positive energy.

Meditation

Meditating is a technique that helps with becoming aware of the things happening around you, the thoughts coming to your mind or concentrating on one thing in order to learn to focus. Scientists have done a lot of studies about meditation and all of them come to the same conclusion that meditation helps with reducing anxiety, sparkling creativity, developing empathy, improving memory, and reducing stress. These are priceless things to obtain for a few minutes devoted to meditation at the beginning of the day.

The most important skill I learned from meditation is understanding that thoughts were like clouds, I could choose to touch them, take them or just let them go. Without practicing this, I do not think I would have been able to understand that I could part from the negative reactions and feelings that I used to have.

Practicing meditation was easy. I used an app to guide me into doing it. Guided meditations made it easy for me to understand how meditation worked.

There is also another kind of meditation that is used by monks. This is the kind where you immerse your mind into thinking about something all day long. It's like when you fall in love and cannot stop thinking about that person. It's the same behavior. Meditating in my mind and longing to receive positive energy will develop the desire in me to practice each of these character traits, building my positive energy to the point that I will change my attitude towards life. And no matter what comes my way, I will be able to face life with confidence, a grateful heart, and a desire to participate fully in the life that was given to me.

Prayer

There are a lot of prayer definitions out there that relate to different dogmas. Which one is the right one? The best definition I can give is that prayer is a relationship of my heart with the Light. In this relationship, I become aware of my strengths and needs and learn to express my gratitude for the life that was given to me. And just like meditation, scientists have discovered that prayer has health benefits and it acts like a mental therapy that promotes healing.

Prayer can be a conversation in my mind, spoken out loud or expressed in writing. No matter what method I choose, at the end of the prayer, the surrender of my spirit and pouring of my heart will be rewarded with peace, hope and every positive energy principle coming from the Light.

In my description of prayer, I would like to highlight what prayer is not. When I started practicing prayer, I used to think that prayer was like talking to a genie. I asked and asked and asked without stopping to think that prayer was more than just asking. One of my spiritual mentors taught me that prayer was a conversation with my higher being. I really did not know what that meant because what kind of conversation can you have with someone you cannot see? How do you start the conversation?

After trying many prayer techniques, I realized how the conversation happen in prayer. It happens by making a connection with my higher being. When I would connect with hope and peace, I felt my spirit connecting with my higher being and I became assured of three things:

- Every single good thing I ever wanted and received comes from the Light.
- The Light does not get separated from me at any point in my life and I do not get separated from the Light at any point in my life either.
- The Light provides me with self-healing and all I need every day of my life.

What these three statements contain is the answer to my need of protection, my need of provision and my need for community. When I feel these needs have been met during my prayer time, my day is peaceful and productive. So, I purposed to obtain these three things through my prayer and meditation time.

When I get up in the morning, the first thing I do is meditate between 10-30 minutes. Then, I purposely center myself to pray for the things I need and want to receive.

The following is an example of one of the meditations I pray in the morning:

Prayer #1

"Light of the World, I thank you for this day. I ask that you fill me up with your energy of gratitude, peace, love, hope, kindness, acceptance, inclusion, self-esteem, forgiveness, healing, happiness, self-control, faith and mercy. I thank you for my healing and the opportunity to enjoy my life fully today. Thank you for teaching me how to rid myself of negative energy, especially fear, anger, shame and guilt. May I be kind to myself, to you and to every being I encounter today. Amen."

Developing a connection with the Light

Having a relationship with the Light may not look like the model some religions use. And if we must compare, the Light is not going to teach you about judging, or avenging, or condemning. A relationship with the Light will do exactly the opposite. You will learn to love yourself and others, to be kind to yourself and others, to seek peace and forgiveness. In this relationship you will also learn about looking at your surroundings, discovering things about yourself, becoming the best version of you.

Every single good thing I ever wanted and received comes from the Light

Let's be honest for a second here. How many times a day do I express my gratitude for having a family, a roof over my head and food on the table? Most likely, not as often as I should. How about being grateful for having life today? I probably do not express my gratitude. We never know what we have until we lose it. I had to learn to become aware of my surroundings and what the Light has provided.

I always say that gratitude is a miracle maker. And in this case the miracle will open your eyes to get to you to know the Light.

When I started to develop my relationship with the Light, I meditated twice a day and prayed in my head all the time. It wasn't because I was infatuated and wanted this relationship. It was because I was in fear and desperate for help. And the more I meditated and prayed for the fear to go away, the more I understood that I needed to change my meditations and prayers. My awareness needed to be on the Light and the positive energy that flows from the Light. I need to concentrate on receiving that positive energy. But instead of opening my hands and my heart to receive it, I was mortified by the power of the negative energy in my life. Little by little, I learned I needed to change the focus of my relationship with the Light. When I stopped concentrating on the negative energy, I found myself being filled with peace.

When I am filled with The Light, I cannot help but to irradiate positivity which will attract all kinds of good things. Positive energy works like math, it is addition, multiplication, abundance, prosperity, healing. In other words, every good thing comes from the Light.

When I started meditating on gratitude and purposely practicing gratitude all day long, it didn't matter if I received bad news, things didn't go my way, or I lost something of value to me. The goal was to be grateful in everything, so I was grateful about my losses and painful events. Because of it, I end up seeing little miracles here and there about how the Light provides for me without me even asking for things.

I remember when I became unemployed. I started to thank the Light for giving me the means to have a roof over my head and food on the table. I literally would meet people who would invite me to lunch or dinner. I understood that having money was not an obstacle for me being fed. When my savings came to an end and I only had one month to pay my mortgage, I decided to sell my condo. For three days I incessantly thanked the Light for allowing me to have lived in my place. I accepted the fact that my unit would no longer be my place and started to make plans to sell it. I also had a hard time finding a job, so I decided to apply for jobs to become an English teacher overseas. It pained me to be grateful, but I did it because I had learned that gratitude would turn into little miracles. And just as I was signing the contracts to get the job overseas and selecting a realtor to sell my condo, a friend of mine told me about a job at his new workplace. The next day, I sent my resume. Then, the following day I went for an interview and in less than 24-hours I had a job offer.

I can't say that I was happy about this job offer. It wasn't the job I wanted. I would be making a lot less money, with a title that was almost an entry level position and with no chances for advancement. I was doubtful if this job was the answer to my prayers. I was used to stressful-managerial jobs that would leave me exhausted and anxious after long-hour days. The job I got was exactly the opposite. I would work my eight hours and then go home.

I knew this was not the job I wanted. But I prayed and asked for the wisdom to know if this was the job I needed. The answer that came was, "I need to be thankful no matter what." I accepted the job.

Being open to the possibility of following a path that didn't necessarily lead me to my desires was a blessing in disguise because it has taught me to be grateful in everything that happens in my life. Gratitude opened my eyes to see my blessings. What I could not see was that I didn't know what I needed, and my expectation was something else. I took the job and with a leap-of-faith I was grateful for having an income, keeping my home, and not moving overseas.

The months passed by and the more I thanked the Light for my job, the more I understood that having the extra time allowed me do things I always dreamed of doing, like writing and photography. Then, several months after I started my job, I found out I had cancer. It was at this moment I understood why I had this job. I had great health insurance and my job allowed me to really take care of myself because I was not tied up in a demanding job. But perhaps one of the biggest blessings of my job was the chance to work with this great gal who became one of my best friends. She was also a cancer survivor as well as a survivor of life. The support that she gave me was incredible and invaluable. I am forever in debt to her for the love and care she extended to me when I needed it the most.

But my biggest blessing for taking this job was the opportunity I had to become closer to my sisters, especially when I found out I had cancer. You see, I was a driven person and didn't really pay attention to family. My sisters went out of their way to take care of me. I do not think I would have had a chance to get closer to them, had I not accepted the job I have today. Had I taken another job, perhaps I would not have slowed down nor had the opportunity to see the healing I received by understanding that family is important because their love was healing to my heart.

I am sure I would not have seen all these blessings, had I not taken the time to be grateful in good times and bad times. Gratitude for me is a miracle maker that helped me trust the Light. This relationship has given me the faith I need to trust that filling myself with the Light and positive energy is a better choice than choosing to listen to negativity, fear, anger and any other negative energy that steals my chances to see a different outcome in my life. I have seen negative energy steal my jobs, my relationships, and my health. Now I know what I must do to keep good things coming into my life.

"Every single good thing comes from the Light" is one of the most essential thoughts I must be aware of when I meditate, when I pray, when I work, and when I live. When I get in the habit of accepting that every good thing comes from the Light, I · realize I also came from the Light. And I am worth receiving good things like love (for myself, for the Light and for every human being on the planet), gratitude, peace, love, hope, kindness, acceptance, inclusion, self-esteem, forgiveness, healing, serenity, happiness (real happiness, not just pleasure), self-control and faith.

The Light does not get separated from me or vice versa

The second thought we must get centered on when we meditate or pray is that we do not get separated from the Light and the Light does not get separated from us because we are light.

The separation I sometimes feel is a deception from negative energy. But as soon as I get rid of any negativity, my spirit understands that I belong to the Light. Knowing that I am light, and *I belong* to the Light changes our view of life.

However, when I am confronted with situations where I feel trapped in a box or I feel angry, then I instantly feel like I am separated, why? Because I have filled up my tank with negative energy. When I do this, then it becomes understandable that I feel separated from the Light. This is why it is so important to be aware of how my mind/soul responds to the events that happen around me.

Scientists have discovered that having negative emotions weaken the immune system. When I think of this in terms of my relationship with the Light, I cannot help but think how I compromised my immune system when I chose not to be in a relationship with the Light. What this says to me is that when I choose to be in a relationship with the Light, I am choosing to love myself.

One of the most wonderful things of being in a relationship with the Light is discovering who I am because my perspective in life changes to reflect the Light. When I discover my skills, abilities, dreams, and passions is like attaining a new lease on life. Understanding this will give me purpose in my daily meditation and prayer and overall in my life.

Every day when I meditate and pray, I must purposely visualize that I am light and I am one with the Light. This is one of the most loving things I do for myself every day. It eases my worries, my fears, my doubts and gives me the strength to ask for more good things for myself like: love (for myself, for the

Light and for every human being on the planet), gratitude, peace, hope, kindness, acceptance, inclusion, self-esteem, forgiveness, healing, serenity, happiness (real happiness, not just pleasure), self-control and faith. These are the things that will help me survive and thrive in life.

The Light provides me with self-healing and all I need

The third thought I must understand and believe in the relationship I develop with the Light is that one of the functions of my body, soul and spirit is self-healing, self-restoration and self-renewal. That's what the Light puts in my system.

This thought is a bit tricky because it requires me to take a leap of faith. However, self-healing and self-restoration are not based on myth, they are based on scientific research and common knowledge that my body heals itself. We do not need a scientist to tell us that when we cut ourselves, our body heals the wound. This is because there is code in our cells and DNA to repair our body. I mention later in this book that DNA repairs itself. The cells in the body also reproduce by mitosis so depending on the part of my body, I can generate new cells in a matter of a few days. So, understanding that I have the capacity to self-heal is not a far-fetch thought. When I am optimistic and full of positive energy, it is easier for my mind, body and spirit to agree that I have the capability to heal and repair and that my self-healing mechanism works.

However, when negative energy lurks around, my spirit feels separated from the Light and my body starts missing the opportunity for self-healing. One example of my self-healing capability being stolen, is fear. When fear enters my mind, my emotions get overwhelmed and my capacity to believe that I will not get sick and/or suffer goes away. This overwhelming feeling makes me feel separated from the Light. And when doubt enters my mind, it truly takes a miracle to go back to believing.

One way to prevent feeling separated from the Light is meditation and prayer. They must be part of our daily routine. Putting it another way, taking the time to make sure I am equipped with the right energy every day is loving myself. Loving myself means that I am willing to sacrifice time and effort to ensure I never forget that I am Light and being light has its benefits if I am filling my tank with positive energy. Having consciousness about our connection to the Light and all the benefits that come from it is winning half the battle when we are faced with doubt, fear, anger, shame, or guilt.

A routine where we include a 10-minute meditation and a 10-minute prayer can do wonders. The meditation can be self-guided. The prayer can be thanksgiving and asking for specific character traits needed to develop a strong bond with the Light. The prayer can also include a request of things we need like health, job security, housing, etc. And we end the prayer time by thanking the Light for providing the things we need.

We must be prepared to say a quick prayer when we feel we are losing our peace. We must always become aware when fear and anger are entering our soul. Usually I speak under my breath a short prayer:

Prayer for Peace:

"Dear Light of the World, please help me be kind, grateful and forgiving. Grant me peace and acceptance of the fact that I cannot change others. And grant me gratitude because you can change my circumstances."

Saying this little prayer when I feel I am being ambushed by fear is like a little jolt of positive energy. It really works because it is an alignment of what I already agreed upon: I am light, and I fill myself up with positive energy. Anything beyond this, does not support me, love me, give me peace, or heal me.

Meditating has allowed me to be aware when negative energy is at my door. It also helps me to practice stopping myself and not allowing myself to lose my peace. Being able to stand my ground and tell fear and anger, "Not today" is one of the most amazing blessings I have received.

It is comforting to know that no matter what comes our way, we have a solution not to feel separated from the Light. Unfortunately, sometimes life throws punches at us and brings us to our knees. Experiencing the loss of a loved one is one of the best examples of this situation. I do not recall any other experience where angst, mixed with the pain felt like a punch to my gut. The grief and pain would not go away. The torment of wanting to go back in time and doing things differently grew stronger with every passing minute because there was no hope to bring the other person back to this realm. Knowing peace and love will bring comfort when loss knocks at my door is a good strategy to have.

So many questions and doubt come to mind when we go through major losses. If this pain is left unattended, the wounds of the spirit and soul become resentment and bitterness. Even if I feel like my loss is an act of injustice and someone has to pay for it, I must love myself above any pain or doubt. If I do not take precautions and this moment takes me by surprise, confusion and fear will automatically take over that part of my brain that makes decisions for me. I must love myself so much that I am prepared not to allow this negative energy to enter my body, soul and spirit. It is at this time when I am most vulnerable that I must recognize and admit that sometimes I cannot make it on my own, especially if my body is going through illness. This is when I need to lean on people to pick me up and carry me when I do not have the strength to do it. This is when I leave my pride behind and ask for help because sometimes it takes a village to see me through.

Walking the walk

It is easy to talk the talk, but it's much harder to walk the walk, especially when the walk is something you were not used to practicing before. I wish I could tell you that it is like doing an exercise program but that would not be accurate because every time I start a fitness program, it becomes a New Year's resolution. By February it is usually an afterthought. Yes, I am that bad when it comes to commitment. But my walk for spiritual fitness is more than a commitment. It is an act of love.

Yes, I am happy to say that my spiritual walk is more than a commitment. It is a demonstration of love for myself. I deserve to be healthy and so do you. What does this love look like? I embrace and accept that I need to respect and be kind to myself to keep me in total health. And as I accept this commitment, I understand I do whatever it takes to achieve it today. Yes, the commitment is just for today (one day at a time) because the present is the only time I have.

Making this commitment makes it easy for me to practice all the activities in my program, especially meditating on the spiritual principles as much as I need them. And the more I practice them, the more energized I feel to go through my day without losing my peace.

A commitment to walk the walk is not a burden when it is motivated by love. Discovering who I am and learning to appreciate myself is the reward I receive when I commit to walking the walk of loving myself.

Walking with the Light

We usually live life without noticing the world around us. Walking with the Light is exactly the opposite. In this walk we are amazed to discover the wonderful world that we live in and not take it for granted. We notice the beauty of the flowers at the park, the awesome singing of the birds in the morning, the contagious laugh of kids, the majesty of the mountains, the charm of a baby, and the love in the eyes of your pet. These are all reasons why we can trust the Light. If life is vibrant and energetic all around us, we can also have that because the source of life is the same, the Light.

Walking with the Light is trusting the positive energy for my well-being, protection, and provision. How does this work? Seeking peace with all people around you will open doors to provide for your needs. Filling yourself with hope will give you favor with the people around you. Being kind to people around you will form a ripple effect that will result in others being kind to you when you need it. And why should we forgive the inexcusable? Because someday we may need forgiveness and the favor will return to us.

The reason to practice all these spiritual principles is not to make me miserable but for me to learn a new way of life where the goal is for me to be healthy, at peace and loving myself and the world around me.

There will always be those moments of disappointment and frustration. And even at those moments there is room to learn new things to understand we do not have to end up disheartened and discouraged because trusting the Light is finding hope for a better tomorrow. All we need today is the strength to walk and trust that the Light will provide us with all we need.

All good things come to those who are willing to walk with the Light and developing a connection with it. Why am I so sure about this? Because positive energy always brings addition, multiplication, prosperity, and health. My life is a witness to all these things.

It takes a village

I am a very independent person. I like finding out how to do things myself because I do not like the ritual that takes place when I have to ask someone to help me. Is this pride? Yes, it is. This need I have to be self-sufficient is based in fear and shame. I do not want anybody to know that I am incapable of doing things myself. But allowing this independence to rule over me has disabled me of the opportunity of others loving me and caring for me. This is why having a village is important. We were created to be social beings and we all need the nurturing found in a village.

We all have different reasons why we choose independence. For me it was because of my experience with my second boyfriend. But to tell you what happened with him, I have to first tell you about my first boyfriend. He was raised in the United States, but his family was from Central America. In his culture, women would let the man make all decisions for them. I was no different from women in his culture. It was nice not to have the responsibility to make decisions. This is why he chose my first car, a car I didn't like but I didn't have the strength to refuse to buy it. The most I could shyly utter was that I didn't like the style. It didn't matter what I said. He took my checkbook and wrote a check and I became the owner of a lemon.

I cannot even begin to recall all the headaches that car gave me. To this day, I do not know if he bought that car to make me dependent on him or if I just got comfortable not dealing with the car issues. Every single time the car broke down, I would be calling him for help. He would fix my car and make me happy. When we broke up I had a rude awakening. No other boyfriend would come to my rescue every time my car broke down.

My second boyfriend was very much the opposite from my first boyfriend. He expected me to meet him halfway in everything. And when my car would break down, he would say: "Call Triple A" or "I don't know what you want me to do. I cannot fix your car." He got so tired of me asking him to do stuff that one day he said to me: "Listen, you are too needy. You need to be more independent." At that very moment I felt like a bucket of iced water was thrown all over me. How dare he call me needy? That evening I went home and decided that nobody would ever call me needy ever again. Hence the reason, I hardly ever ask for help now.

Fast forward to when I started my healing journey, my counselor told me I needed to build my village. I thought that was a suggestion, so I didn't do it. He kept insisting that I do it, so I started to look for support groups that didn't require a commitment. But once I started to attend, I felt the good it was doing to my soul to know that I was not alone dealing with my loneliness. I kept going because I wanted to hear more about how to get out of the funk.

When I was diagnosed with cancer, I knew I could not deal with it on my own. The future was too dark, my legs were literally shaky, and I felt like someone needed to carry me. I remembered all those times I felt invincible, like nothing was going to stop me. And now, I was standing at a fork in the road. One choice was to try to deal with the sickness, surgery and treatment on my own. The second one was to ask for help. I do not know what hurt more, admitting that I was human or asking for help. But the combination felt like a big blow to my ego. I am grateful that I opted for the latter.

I am the fourth of eight children in my family and the oldest sister. I have a very strong drive so when I finished high school, I had a list of things I wanted to accomplish, including attending college very far away from home. This list made me become a stranger to my family. I was all about work and accomplishing goals. I never had the need to get to know my own family because I was too busy trying to build a career. When I had the need to build a village to help me through my recovery from cancer, I wasn't quite sure if any of my siblings would be willing to go through it with me.

Getting sick was a blessing in disguise because I had to slow down and look around to see what really mattered. What I saw was my family, my two sisters and their big hearts and how unselfish they were. Even though I had never been there for them, they did not hesitate to be there for me when I told them about my diagnosis. The one sister who lives an hour from me, opened up her home and without reservation or asking for anything in return took me in and cared for me until I could go back to work. She and her husband gave me anything I needed. At that time my other sister was visiting my sister with whom I was staying and between the two of them, they fed me, tucked me into bed, woke up three times during the night every night to take me to the bathroom, and the list goes on and on. This love I would have never felt or experienced if I hadn't made the choice to ask for help.

The other blessing, I received with my diagnosis was the revelation that my persona in social media was not the village my counselor told me to build. My social media persona had thousands of friends, but I didn't have a clue how to truly connect with people. In order to really reach out to people, I had to turn off the social media persona and let the real me walk into my life. I was blessed I found friends who were willing to walk with me and to hold my hand. One in particular, who lives 2,500 miles from me and in a different time zone, took the time to call me, text me every day before my surgery and all the way through my recovery. She went shopping online for my needs. She made sure I had everything I needed. We had been friends for a very long time but when I moved to another state, we couldn't help but fall apart. I thought I would never find another friend like her and to be honest, I didn't want to bother finding anybody else like her. When my heart became bare and I found myself wanting someone in my time of need, this lovely friend came to mind.

Baring my heart and my situation to her over the phone I asked her to be with me through it all and she did. Our bond was intense, it felt like she was in the same room with me wherever I went. Being close to her not only brought happiness but also healing to my life.

Opening my heart for the first time in a long time and standing there being vulnerable felt like offering my heart. I didn't know how much time left I had so I had to approach life in a different way. Sharing my heart was a chance I took to offer love in exchange for love. The response I received was overwhelming because I didn't believe people would extend their love to me. I thought I didn't need anyone, but the fact was I was hungry and thirsty for love, nonetheless my approach to get it was completely wrong. The people that cared for me wanted my heart, not my accomplishments, or my looks. And the funniest part was that I wanted the same. Having this revelation was like finding love, a love I lost and was happy to rediscover.

I cannot say enough about my support groups and how they have affected my healing journey. It was in these groups that I learned I was not alone. I also discovered that I could share in confidence the secrets of my heart that were causing me pain. I learned to become a social being. It was here where I found my second family. I also found my higher being that did not judge me. And I thankfully uncovered the sanity that I did not know I was missing. And when I was diagnosed with cancer, it was there that I found catharsis, a purging of my fears and anger for being sick, and gratitude for being given the gift of life.

I also have to give credit to my counselor. He took the time to peel off all the layers of denial, fear, anger, shame and guilt and taught me about "responsibility." I was very good at playing the victim and never thought I needed to take responsibility for allowing negative energy into my body. I was not guilty or responsible about other people's behavior, but I was responsible about taking care of my body, keeping my mind's sanity and feeding my spirit the right kind of energy. I was not doing that because I was keeping resentment and allowing self-hatred to dwell in my mind and body. Learning about taking responsibility was the best investment I made in myself.

I can't complete my village record without mentioning my spiritual mentor. He was like a father to me who taught me to sweep the floors of my mind and wash the walls of my spirit. He taught me about prayer and healing. He taught me to believe that coincidences could be miracles, answers to my prayers. He taught me that I was a wonderful human being and my mistakes of the past should not define my future. His support and mentoring were invaluable and indescribable. He was the father figure I never had, and I always felt protected whenever I was in his presence. I didn't know these were things parents would give their children. I am profoundly grateful that I learned about and received this protection even when I was an adult.

The other spiritual mentors that came after my first one taught me about the great benefits of meditating, listening, using creativity as a way of healing, loving myself, getting out of my cocoon and enjoying myself in any situation. They taught me to discover the world around me with new eyes. My perception of the world had trapped me in the negative perceptions I had. It was my spiritual mentors who liberated me from my own bounds and taught me to look at the things that were important. I am forever grateful for their influence on me. They helped set me free. And I can say without hesitation that freedom from my own preconceptions never felt so good.

I also have a spiritual community as in a religious organization. When I gather in this group, I make sure that the people I relate to, seek the same goals as I do, to fill myself up with love, peace, kindness, forgiveness, gratitude, faith and the like as a primary motive. I do this because sometimes the primary purpose of a religious group is to preserve rituals. I do not say this lightly and I do not mean to bash religion, but the activities and rituals of religion are important but not as important as making sure I am filled with positive energy which is my most important goal in life. I do not take lightly getting sick and developing mental conditions. This is why my most important priority is to love myself by filling up my body, soul, and spirit with positive energy. Does this sound selfish? It might, but when I consider the outcome will be showing kindness, gentleness, gratitude, love, and peace to the world, I'd say this is the kind of self-consideration that I need and must have.

In my village, I also got some other experts like a doctor, a nutritionist, fitness trainer, food experts and healers who share their knowledge with me and encourage me. I had to get rid of my disliking of going to the doctor. I go see my primary doctor regularly. I have chosen one who listens to me and keeps an open mind to alternative medicine and guides me when and how to take the path of holistic medication. I take medication prescribed by my doctor, but I believe that what I put in my mouth to eat is my primary medicine. This is why my diet consists primarily of vegetables and fruits. I have a friend who is my fitness trainer, she helps me maintain an exercise program. For the most part, my exercise program consists of walking every day for 30 minutes. I walk and make sure I do it every day because fitness and staying active help me get a grip on stress. Staying active also helps me keep my mind sharp and helps me sleep better. Whenever I have questions about my health, I ask my group of experts in my village to make educated decisions.

For all these reasons, I procured a village to raise me from physical illnesses, loneliness and suffering. They are the ones who lift me up when I need it. Building a village is perhaps one of the best gifts I gave myself. The community I built around myself has become a shield when I can't see the danger I am putting myself into.

Putting myself in danger is indulging in erratic behavior; like being irresponsible and going out when the government is asking me to stay at home due to a pandemic. Putting my health in danger and the health of others just because I felt that the rules didn't apply to me is definitely not loving myself. Being kind to me reflects on me being kind to others. So, when my mind thinks I'm having an adventure when it's clearly not, then I must listen to my village.

Thinking only of myself and not being kind has consequences. I may not see them right away, but they may be obvious when I need help, and nobody steps forward to do it.

Having a village will guide me and teach me to be considerate of myself and others. A village will show me how to love myself and others. A village will forgive my mistakes and instill in me the desire to forgive others so I can learn to let go of my anger. A village will demonstrate how to heal so I can go and do the same with others in need. In doing so, I will learn to love unconditionally. A village will give me hope that I am not alone in my healing journey. For all these reasons, building a village is a sign of loving myself.

One thing I made sure while I was building my village was to minimize my contact with people who had negative energy because dark energy is contagious. I avoid engaging my energy with theirs, but I always bless them. I choose every day to be around people who have the same goals and desires as me: to love myself, to heal myself, to keep myself healthy, sane, and strong. Loving life is a sign of loving myself and I want to do this to the best of my abilities.

Making a commitment to love myself

What is the conclusion of this chapter? I must make a commitment to only allow positive energy in my life. Why should I bother with positive energy? Why should I follow a program designed to receive positive energy? The answer is very simple. Because I want to learn a new way of loving myself.

For some reason, the phrase "making a commitment" sounds hard to do. The thoughts that come to mind are, "I don't have enough time as it is." And my response to those thoughts are: "I deserve being loved by me."

Love is not just a feeling; it is a spiritual principal that brings healing to the world. Love is the force that gives me the power to be kind, forgiving, accepting, creative, loving, and so many more positive qualities. If love is part of the positive package, I want to make a commitment to love myself.

But before we go into the spiritual program, we need to understand how my spirituality relates to my body. By appreciating how we connect to the light, we are going to take a trip into science and learn about the most important part in us: our human spirit. Yes, science little by little is making the connection between our body and spirituality. Let's take a look.

Chapter 4

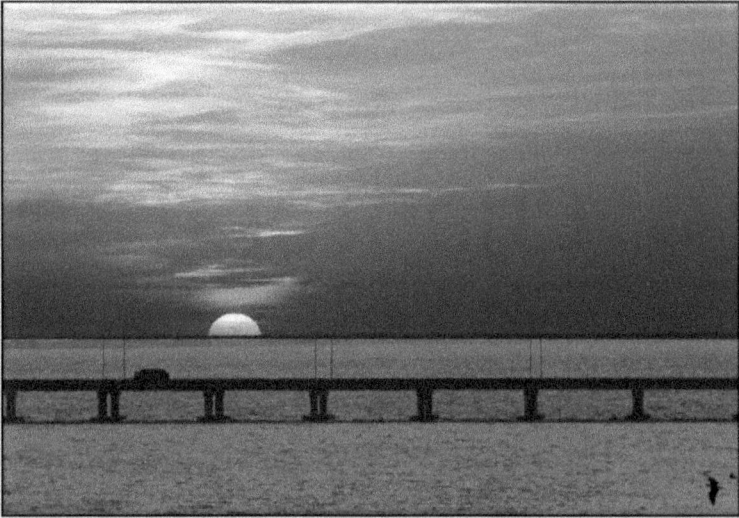

Where Science Meets Spirituality

S cience does not support anything that cannot be proven. And spirituality is considered a personal experience that connects you to a higher consciousness. This consciousness is not the reptilian brain but the mind that makes the right choices like choosing to love over accepting fear because you trust in a higher being.

What is the connection between science and spirituality? They seem to be as far as the East is from the West. But when we think about healing, science is discovering that our body is equipped for self-healing. So praying and meditating for our body to heal is not a far fetch idea because our bodies are equipped to do it and our body, soul and spirit just need to be infused with the right energy to do so. I would like to start this chapter with a couple of examples about the job of electricity in our body.

The first example is Bioelectricity, a sub-discipline of biology that studies the electrical currents in our bodies. Electricity is how the neurons in the brain communicate to the cells in the rest of the body. The most recent studies of bioelectricity have found that slow currents in the cells produce a slower healing time in the body. Changing the current in the cells can accelerate the healing of the organs.

Currently there are several studies being conducted to study the relation between cancer and the electrical currents in the cells. The theories basically say that the electrical currents carrying instructions to the cells being developed cannot communicate correctly causing the developing cells to mutate. These same studies are looking for the right treatment with electricity that will allow the cell to open up and link to the correct communication and in turn heal the cells.

The second example is a great discovery that geneticists have done in the last few years. DNA must replicate in our bodies because it allows for cell division. Without this replication, our cells cannot carry the genetic characteristics or create the proteins needed for the cells to survive. The replication of DNA doesn't come without issues. When the process of replication becomes unstable, our DNA strands get damaged or mutated causing aging and diseases. The older we get, the more unstable this process becomes. When DNA has to repair itself, geneticists have discovered that certain enzymes attach to the DNA to repair the strands. However, these enzymes render ineffective when they are ionized with too much phosphate (charged with the wrong electricity). But when the enzymes are charged correctly, the DNA can bind and repair. In other words, geneticists have pinpointed to an electric charge as being responsible to glue the DNA strands and heal them when they get damaged.

These two fantastic discoveries in science are changing the way we look at electricity in our bodies. I am not a biologist or a geneticist, but I can see that the atoms on earth and in the universe are guided by energy, so are the most intricate parts of heredity, cell replication and healing of life.

What I see in these science examples is that every breath of life is because the electric charges and currents produce life in me. My body grows and my cells reproduce because the electricity I need is there to guide my body how to do it. Having the right energy circulating in my body, soul and spirit will increase my health.

But where does this electricity come from? What is its origin? Science cannot tell us yet where it comes from. Not meaning to be a hater here, but while science catches up, I am going to fill out the blanks about this electricity that I call the Light and the positive energy that flows from it. The following chapters are about the connection between the Light with our body, soul/mind and spirit. And the positive energy that emanates from the Light to give us life and health.

But before we get into it, let's revisit some concepts that we will need to see how the Light affects all of us.

The realms of my existence

I am not just body; I also have a soul and a human spirit.

I am three parts: body, soul, and spirit

I know everyone is aware of these concepts. My desire for this section is not to bore you with something that you already know. I am going through my own descriptions because my views come from a mixture of science and spirituality. I would not have put them in here if they were not important. Please read with an open mind as if you are learning about them for the first time.

A human being is composed of three parts. Body, soul and spirit. All three parts go through a phase of development and learning. Then, a human being goes through a period of thriving and reproduction. In the older days, the body sees the effects of aging. And just as the physical body needs different foods and exercises at different phases of its life, the soul and spirit need feeding and support, especially when a person suffers losses in her/his life.

So, buckle up and let's engage in a new way of seeing our soul and human spirit. I promise it; it will be worthwhile.

Body

The body is the physical side of our beings. It's not difficult to recognize it because it is the most comprehensive, limited part of who we are. The body is an amazing resilient machine that runs automatically. It heals or repairs itself and has alarms that notify the body to grow, to stop body development and to cease certain functions when they are no longer needed. Who directs and gives our body the guidance needed to function without a hitch? For the most part, it is our soul or mind.

Soul or Mind

In this book, the soul is not described as what's taught in many dogmas as the immortal part of a human being. This book takes a scientific point of view to define how the soul works. Describing what the soul covers is a bit more ambiguous than the body because we cannot see the whole extent of it. It is not really palpable although it has a big job: to take care of our body and make sure everything runs without a glitch. In order to do this, the soul encompasses three big areas: Consciousness or mind, emotions and decision making.

It is not an accurate example to equate our soul/mind to a computer but everything that happens in the mind can be compared to algorithms, processes, and memory that a computer needs to run. The processes involved in managing our body are called "synaptic connections." These are electric impulses (electricity) that carry on execution programs to operate, maintain, feed, protect, heal and do whatever it takes to keep up our bodies in top shape.

It hasn't been until recently that scientists have admitted that consciousness has a bigger role than what they were willing to admit. Science has not made a connection yet between consciousness and the millions of synaptic connections happening in the neurons, nor how the brain makes a trillion decisions a day for us without missing a heartbeat. All these electrical connections firing a trillion times a day are still, for the most part, a mystery to science and therefore to all of us.

However, science can now identify the parts of the brain involved in the functions of the body. An example of this is when the body is in pain or when a person is feeling pleasure. It just so happens that these electric impulses firing in the brain are responsible for the brain recognizing pain and pleasure. But at the same time, science cannot differentiate which is the electric signal that signifies pain, or which is the one that signifies pleasure. What this means is that the "code" that the brain sends as a command when I am in pain or when I am feeling pleasure is not known yet. To understand better, let's see a couple of examples:

Example number one: The nerves send a signal to my brain when I burn my fingers on the stove and in return my brain sends me the awareness that I have been injured and registers that as pain. All of these messages are communicated by the brain with electrical impulses.

Example number two: My eyes are looking at the exquisite aqua-blue water of the ocean and the white sugary sands. My optical nerves send the signal to the brain and in turn, the brain registers this experience and sends an electric impulse letting me know that I am having a delightful, pleasurable experience.

Even though those are two completely different experiences and one causes me pain and the other pleasure, all science knows at the moment is that the communication between my body and my mind is in the form of electrical impulses or electrical signals. And even though scientist can track these electric impulses from my nerves to different parts of the brain and vice versa, scientist cannot tell the difference about what synaptic connections have the code of pain, and which ones have the code of pleasure or happiness.

Deciphering the code of these electrical impulses is one of the most important functions of the soul. Overseeing every single aspect of our bodies is the job of the soul. As mentioned before, there are three areas involved in managing the body: consciousness or the mind, emotions and decision making.

Consciousness

It is defined by many psychologists, scientists, and philosophers as that state of awareness where the mind registers everything that happens including the functioning of the body, thinking process, recording of emotions and decisions that our mind makes.

Without a doubt, our mind is a big computer processor that makes a zillion recordings of all that enters into our awareness through the senses and not only registers everything but also makes decisions to keep the body going. Among those decisions, the mind sends signals to the body for optimal functioning, self-growing, self-healing, problem solving, recalling memories, learning, enjoying an activity, etc. This list goes on and on and happens thanks to the trillions of synaptic connections that the neurons have on a given day. Thanks to our consciousness, we experience life and register these experiences and sort them out.

Emotions

According to social sciences, emotions are a mental state as a result of behavioral responses to experiences, feelings, physiological responses to events happening inside or outside our bodies.

Unlike body functions, I believe emotions are ruled not only by our mind but also by the seed of our emotions sitting in our guts and heart. This is why when we have emotional pain, we may perceive the pain in our chest; therefore, we call it a "broken heart." This is also why a person feels "butterflies" in the stomach when they are falling in love.

There is also that saying, "I have a gut feeling," when a person refers to perceptions that are not rational but come from emotional discernment in our gut. They may be conscious or subconscious associations of experiences from the past that have influenced the seed of our emotions in our gut and therefore, influence the outcome of our decisions in the future.

The gut-brain connection is not a myth. There are scientific studies with evidence that the gastrointestinal track is attuned to our emotions. Some scientific journals go on to say that the gut is our second brain. Some research studies say that rational thinking and decision making come from the brain. But when it comes to emotional thinking and decision making, it comes from our gut.

Why is this fact important? Because mental health issues are very much connected to the health of the gastrointestinal track. Strong emotions are felt in the gut. And what are these emotions? Anger, stress, anxiety, depression, just to mention a few, are emotions that are felt in the gut and scientific studies confirm that they affect the digestive system and vice versa.

One of the primary functions of emotions is decision making. Which means that for every decision we make, not only the brain is involved but also an emotional consideration. Let me say this again, every decision we make has an emotion attached to it. Going to college, choosing a career, choosing a partner in life, even what time we go shopping has an emotion attached to it. This is why keeping our soul healthy makes for the best decisions we can make.

Decision making

The third main function of the soul is our decision making. Just like computer programming would function, when we are in the learning phase of our life, our mind and emotions form code about our preferences and the next time we come across the same decision, we already have an algorithm in our decision-making part of the soul/mind that helps with time management.

Once our decision making becomes automatic, it can be classified as behavior. The same can be said about our brain processing information in a nano second that results in strong emotions to events happening in our awareness.

The reptilian brain resides in the decision-making part of the mind, where the self-preservation behavior is deployed automatically. This is why our body responds automatically to decisions concerning feeding, fighting, fleeing and reproduction. We still can stop these decisions, but it takes self-control, a higher consciousness of the brain to stop these decisions.

For example, if I am taking a walk in the woods and come across a mountain lion, my instinct will tell me to flee immediately. This primal instinct to flee danger is a result of my reptilian brain. This decision involves a state of mind (emotion) and my consciousness' response to it, without me being conscious of making a decision. But in less than a second, my instinct makes the decision to flee from the danger I am encountering. There are other decisions I make that come to my awareness and I consciously make an effort to decide. An example of this, is when I choose what I am going to wear to go to work. I believe this "decision making" is part of a learning process and once I decide what the appropriate attire to go to work is, my mind learns the "algorithm" of "work clothes." Once the code is registered in my mind, it doesn't take me as much time each day to decide what I am going to wear. I, more or less, subconsciously buy clothes that fit my profile of "work clothes" and all of sudden, my attempts to choose my work wardrobe are effortless because I already figured out the "algorithm" in my head.

My choices for the decisions I make every day, are basically tied to behaviors that are some form of algorithm in my mind. Once the behavior is formed, my mind does not have to repeatedly formulate my decisions. They are stored in my subconscious mind and brought to my consciousness automatically. This is why advertisers are personalizing more and more ads that we see on our smart phones, tablets and streaming services. All the data that we leave behind is the behavior or our own "algorithm" that can pinpoint our preferences and habits involved when we buy online.

The soul or mind is one of the most amazing works of engineering and art. Its work is so seamless and subtle, that we do not realize its complexity and virtuosity. I do not want to give scientist a bad rap about anything because thanks to them we have advanced so much. But also, I must say that for hundreds of years, scientists have not recognized the soul (consciousness or mind, emotions and "decision making") as a crucial component of the human body because as explained before, it is not yet understood how the electrical signals carry the "code" to keep us alive, safe and healthy. I hope more and more scientists discover the wonders of the soul.

Having said this, I think we need to give the soul (consciousness, emotions and decision making) room to be recognized as a fundamental part of the operating system of our body. Just because we have not been able to identify the full function of our soul, it doesn't mean that we must disregard the miracle of having a well-run machine that is capable of storing and developing memories, emotions, feelings, and decisions just to mention a few.

In physics there is a theory called Quantum Entanglement that can relate to the soul's operating system and this can be even more visible when it comes to collective consciousness. Quantum entanglement is the theory that was first proposed by physicists and explained by Einstein as the "spooky action at a distance" when two photons (particles of light) were linked and mirroring each other regardless of the space between them. This behavior could describe the mind's behavior when a person is in chaos in their mind and meditates and take deep breaths. Little by little the afflicted mind starts mirroring the peace entering the body and calms down. There is an agreement in your soul sent to all cells in your body to release any thoughts of worry and anxiety and it is done so. In other words, unity is found in the soul and it unites the body to follow the decision of the mind by mirroring the energy that enters the body.

The Quantum Entanglement theory is exemplified when the collective consciousness of scientists starts mirroring knowledge and putting it to work. This is why the scientific community has advanced so much in technology, medical procedures, engineering, social sciences and in every area of science because the scientific community has been passionate about finding answers and solutions and the knowledge mirrors everywhere, causing unity for advances in technology.

The Quantum Entanglement theory is also demonstrated when the collective consciousness helps someone in distress and a group of people come to an agreement to help the person in affliction. Whether the help comes in the form of prayer, finances, moral support or any other way, the person in affliction attains confidence and "faith" that the solution that they cannot bring by themselves, can be found with the support of others. In this example, there is this positive energy of agreement that changes the point of view of the afflicted person from negative to positive. The same can be said of negative energy. A group of people can be content at work but a single person going around and complaining about the work conditions can bring doubt and dissatisfaction that will spread around like a fire.

Another example the behavior of Quantum Entanglement is the flu or COVID 19. One single person can bring the virus to a place and the virus will mirror itself or spread like fire, making a lot of people sick. Why give this example of an illness? Illness is a form of negative energy that depletes the sources of positive energy in the body and the ability to keep healthy. When negative energy enters the body like a virus, it will start mirroring it in the entire body and all of a sudden, four days later you are in bed sick.

It is my hope that we will continue to understand the soul (consciousness, emotions and "decision making") and thrive to discover its amazing functions.

And as we discover how important the soul is, we also become aware that just as the body, our soul needs care in order to function well. Our soul must be fed and maintained just as the body is. As the operating system, my soul is also susceptible to viruses. It is my job to provide for an antivirus program. When the soul or our operating system is not well, we see the symptoms that affect the mood, thinking and behavior of a person. Soul maintenance is a topic that will be addressed in the following chapters.

Spiritual Realm

We are now entering an area that is believed to be mysticism. For centuries, the spiritual realm has been a mysterious subject. Science has denied the existence of it because there is no way to prove it exists. The idea of a god and a spiritual realm comes from religion. For centuries, religions have based their beliefs on the existence of God and have given their explanation as to how the universe was formed, where we come from, how life began in this planet and the purpose of our being. Most religions teach of God as a ruler of the spirits or spiritual realm and the earth being under the control of the spiritual realm. Depending on the religion, God may be denoted as the Divine, the Universe, the Enlightenment, and or the Light.

This section is about the spiritual world and how humanity fits in it. Spirituality in this book is not about siding with one religion or advocating for a specific divinity.

The explanation of the Light in this book is about looking into nature, what we have discovered and understanding what is missing and filling in the blanks. We all come from and are attached in every way to the Light. Yes, we are a progeny of the Light and our bodies, as well as the earth and the universe. We behave the same way as the atomic world that quantum physics and quantum mechanics have tried to explain for the last century. Out of all the theories that science has come up with about the beginning of the universe, I like the M-theory the best because it describes the structure and behavior of our bodies.

In a few words, the M-theory basically says that there are dimensions that can be unified with the elements of spacetime and gravity by declaring that all dimensions are one dimension attached to a second dimension acting as a 'membrane.' To see it in a different way, the subatomic elements hang together thanks to a membrane that wraps them all. The model of the substructure of subatomic particles is the model that we can see in other parts of the universe like the ecosystem in my body or the ecosystem on earth.

The main components of my body are oxygen and hydrogen (water) and my body is home to trillions of bacteria, viruses and fungi in my intestines, my mouth, on my skin and pretty much every part of my body. These microbes help me digest food, keep me healthy and support my survival. There is a mutual understanding that I help the microbes exist and they do the same for me. They form colonies to defend me and keep me healthy from any other harmful bacteria or overpopulation of harmful bacteria.

This amazing ecosystem that I carry around and all my organs that offer housing to the microbes are bound by one membrane: my skin. Just like the description of the M-theory, my skin is a membrane where organisms smaller than my organs are attached and are enclosed by my skin making it one unit that makes me unique and makes me…me!

The same concept applies to the atomic world. For example, hydrogen particles are very flammable. When hydrogen reacts and releases a photon (electric charge), it loses electrons. Instead of becoming a new element, it gathers new electrons to become the old hydrogen it used to be. The hydrogen particle isn't confused about what it is. No matter how many electrons it loses or gains, it goes back to be what it was meant to be.

I propose that all atomic particles as well as my body act just as the hydrogen particle. No matter what changes I go through, at the end my identity is the same. I remain the same as the atoms inside of me because there is code inside of me that keeps me being a unit, just like the atomic elements carry code to remain what they are supposed to be, a unique unit to function for the purpose it was created.

Just like the code in my DNA that describes what color of eyes I have, my height, the color of my hair, etc., everything that exists in the universe carries a code that executes to keep us functioning as intended. It's like some sort of glue that keeps my microbes and organs inside of my skin, keeping the design in which, I was created. We already know that my DNA is code inside of me that describes who I am from the minute I was conceived. I believe it is the same for the rest of the world and the universe. That code that is executed via electric charges belongs to the Light. And that electromagnetism that carries the waves of electricity is the Light.

A very interesting fact that proves my point is the fact that my microbiome (the microbe colonies in my body) is unique to me, just like my fingerprints or the iris of my eye or the vibrations of energy I emit. Science agrees and has proven that all these things are unique to each individual.

Why am I highlighting this fact? Because when I look at the earth, I can see the same pattern. She is an ecosystem. She also has a main composition element: oxygen. Water covers about seventy percent of the surface of earth helping produce five kingdoms of life: bacteria, algae, fungi, plants and animals. To name all species in each kingdom would take an encyclopedia but enough to say that the earth is home to in infinite number of living things. That is the code of the earth, to produce life, all kinds of life no matter the terrain or type of weather. And all of them carrying their own code to make them unique, a unit that functions as they were meant to be.

Our planet is unique in every single way. No planet in the solar system can claim to have such a unique variety of living things even though life has been discovered in other planets. The earth can be described as a "greenhouse" because the atmosphere covers the earth like skin or a membrane, just like the M-theory describes the sub-atomic particles or strings being surrounded with a membrane. That is similar to our body being surrounded by a membrane called skin.

Our planet earth is unique in every way and the same can be said of the planets in our solar system. None of the planets seem like earth even though there are chemical elements that are the same. Each planet in our solar system seems to be unique. The same can be said about the universe, even though we do not have all facts. However, pictures of the Hubble telescope have captured the spectacular story that each galaxy is unique and different just like our milky way and our solar system. And what seems to be the element that surrounds the universe like a membrane? I am going to take a wild guess that dark matter is the membrane of the universe. But what is the element that unites us all and makes us be from the same fabric? The Light, that electromagnetic vibration that exists everywhere and carries the code and commands to make us all unique and very much spectacular.

Because of all these reasons, without a doubt, I can call the Light a higher being because it's the essence in all matter (alive and inanimate). No matter where I go or what I do, I cannot escape the fact that energy and the traces of its essence make me who I am so in a sense everything is a derivative and creation of the Light. I know this because the smallest part of me is the atom and atoms are energy and energy is light. The same can be said about the universe because science has discovered that the smallest components of the universe are atomic particles in atoms which means the universe is also made from Light. This energy that is captured in our bodies is what gives us life. The fuel and commands that make my soul or mind manage my body to function properly comes from and is Light.

The Light - the Spirit of Life

The Light is the source of all matter and life; and the source of all positive energy. One of the purposes of this writing is to propose that the Light possess the characteristics of what we would consider to be God: omnipresence, omnipotent and omniscient. Why are these the characteristics of God? Because they comprise the knowledge and consciousness to produce all kinds of life. And this life manifests as the "energy" or Light that flows in all of us that we received when we are conceived.

One may say that conviction is needed to make that leap of faith and to accept that the Light is indeed that higher being. Especially when science will not accept any hypothesis unless there is a way to prove it. And I respond with a question. How does science explain that sparkle of energy that enters the ovule and sperm when a woman conceives and makes the starting point of life? Or how does science explain the ending of life when that sparkle of energy leaves the body and a person takes their last breath? What is that energy in the heart that makes it pump blood? Or the energy that brings oxygen and nutrients to every organ of the body through the blood? Or that energy that triggers the electrical connections firing in the brain a trillion times a day? Or why meditation improves the immune system and reduces blood pressure? Or how forgiveness improves mental health, heart health and reduces anxiety and stress? Or how peace of mind heals the brain? Or how hope reduces physical pain and improves cardiovascular health? The list of all the benefits of the positive energy of the Light are countless.

Just because we cannot explain how it works, it doesn't mean that the Light does not exist or its involvement. One amazing fact is that the brain uses twenty percent of the energy in the body. And one-quarter of this energy is utilized by the glial cells and neurons to maintain and support homeostasis, the process that keeps a person alive. The other seventy-five percent is used to create electrical charges from the brain to all the cells in the body and vice-versa. What this means is that the electricity or energy in our body is what keeps us alive. In other words, this energy is the spirit of life.

There is no science book at this time that can explain where this amazing Light or "energy" comes from or how it works. Nonetheless, this will not stop the Light from doing what it has been doing for zillions of years, which is producing life, healing, and restoring.

The Light is such force that no science, religion, or human being can utterly and absolutely comprehend or explain it to the full agreement of humanity. But what nobody can deny is that on earth, living things and inanimate objects are ruled and governed by those electromagnetic waves called the Light. Yes, the foundation of our beings according to quantum physics is electromagnetic fields of light and as such, we are a derivative and creation of this amazing energy called Light.

This energy is what I call the spiritual realm that manifests as a network of electrical connections that unites us all in some manner. All matter is connected and part of this energy that is the code of life. For a lack of a better example, the Light is executable code like in a computer that is carried out in all matter. This code, energy or Light is the life emanating from me. It is what forms life and gives me knowledge. Its presence is felt in every single corner of the universe. This is why the Light is omnipotent, omniscient and omnipresent.

Omnipotent

The Light is omnipotent (all power) because it has the power to produce life, create anything, and make everything that exists in the universe, things that are known and unknown. It has the power to change the state of elements on earth like the water becoming solid as ice, gas as vapor or liquid as water. It has the power to give life to an ovule and a sperm when a woman conceives or take life away when a person dies. The Light has the power to infuse peace of mind when we meditate. The Light has the power to remove anxiety, depression, pain, and speed healing if we infuse ourselves with love. The Light has the power to drive out fear when we let love be the ruler of our heart.

Omniscient

The Light is omniscient (all knowledge) because it carries the code of all knowledge and brings it into everything that is in existence. An example of this is our DNA, the code that executes when we are conceived and determines our sex, eye color, hair color, longevity, impulsive tendencies, etc. Another example is musical notes. When musical notes have certain arrangement and hit certain tones that express sadness, my mood can change by listening to that music because my emotions are programmed to become sad when I hear those tones and the vibrations of music hit my body and emotions. Another example is the way our eyes register the colors when the light hits an object. This is how we are able to describe the colors. A person who is color blind cannot register in their brain the colors because that code or knowledge does not exist in their brain. The previous water example is perfect to describe knowledge or code in the water. For instance, the water changes into solid when the temperature goes below 32° Fahrenheit, so the code in water basically says that if the temperature changes when water is present, the water will be affected by those changes. When the temperature reaches 212° Fahrenheit, the code in water makes water change into gas or vapor. And water becomes liquid when the temperature is above 32° Fahrenheit. This code or knowledge in water cannot be seen, nonetheless, it exists, and it doesn't matter what we do or say or ignore about this code, it will trigger and execute when certain conditions apply.

Omnipresent

The Light is omnipresent (present everywhere) because the electromagnetic waves that form all substance is found in all matter (alive and inanimate); this includes all beings and inanimate objects on earth and the universe. This energy is in constant movement within our bodies and around us.

Everything that exists in this world functions because of the presence of the Light in them. Having the presence of the Light, or this energy in us is vital for our survival. And this energy is what connects us to everyone and everything on earth.

Just like the sun, the Light brings sunlight to the earth. This metaphor is the understanding that the Light is the energy that brings life, hope, prosperity, and enlightenment to this world. This is the reason why I sometimes call it "The Light of this world."

Human Spirit

In physics, light is described as a particle and waves. Physicists also have discovered in recent years that people are waves, referring to the ability to absorb or reject energy, with unique frequencies. My understanding of this is that the vibrations or waves of energy that I emit, are unique to me as if it were a fingerprint. This unique light within me that regulates my heartbeat, my blood flow, my respiratory movements, is my human spirit that connects with other human beings and the rest of the universe. In other words, I am light.

My human spirit, or my own brand of energy, is what gives me life. And just as the Light possesses the ability of power, knowledge and presence, so does my human spirit but at an individual level which is what makes me unique in every single sense of the word.

Human Power

My human spirit gives me the capability of power to create, to build, to destroy, to love, to have power over people, etc. This power is charged by the energy that I exude. My energy gives me power to achieve goals and persevere. And just as I can be filled with positive energy and do great things, I can also be filled with negative energy and destroy others as well as myself. The power in me is like a vessel that I can infuse with positive energy (love) or negative energy (fear).

Human Knowledge

There are two parts to the human knowledge. First part is the innate knowledge part. It's inside of me like a code that my body receives the instant I am conceived. An example of the innate knowledge is the behavior of the fertilized egg or zygote that follows the embryogenesis development where cells begin to divide, and implantation of the embryo occurs in the uterus. This knowledge is a miracle where the zygote innately knows that the only way to survive is by the cells multiplying themselves in the uterus. Another example of innate knowledge is procreation where humans feel the urge to procreate when their bodies become suitable for procreation and the hormones innately work to make the body ready for the possibility of conception. Scientists classify this code as the reptilian brain.

The second part of human knowledge doesn't need much explanation. Life is a learning process where parents teach the toddler to walk, to talk and to behave. Then comes school (all levels) to teach a person about society, the sciences, the environment, and life. The learning process goes beyond school and extends as a life learning experience. This knowledge is my capacity of learning through the years.

Human Presence

The presence part of my human spirit is, in my opinion, what people call "first impressions," formed by that energy that I exude. This reminds me of what the philosopher Rene Descartes said: "I think, therefore I am" or "I exist, therefore, I am." As simple as this phrase, my human spirit is the reason why I exist.

All of us in this universe are autonomous but best function when we come together and act in agreement to bring ourselves as a vessel of this higher being's energy that gives us life and purpose. Without going into philosophical or theological debates, because there are none to bring to the table, I call this energy "the Light" because this is the universal symbol of hope, life, enlightenment, power and infinite source of energy.

It is mind blowing when I think about how The Light manifests in my life through my human spirit giving me what I need to be alive. Without this energy, my body is just inanimate matter. This sparkle of life that travels throughout my body is my human spirit being in charge of this amazing work of engineering called my body and soul or mind. And just as a car needs refills on gas, so does my human spirit. Recharging my human spirit is what I do when I sleep, meditate, pray and any activity that fills my body with positive energy.

But life is not as simple as just me putting gas in the car. This magnificent work of art that I carry around and manage has the capacity to recharge with two types of fuel: positive energy and negative energy. The latter energy does not give me life, build me up or cause me to prosper. Negative energy does exactly the opposite. It takes away my life, my health, my hopes, my dreams, and pretty much everything that I have. More about dark energy in the following chapters. But first let's talk about total health.

Chapter 5

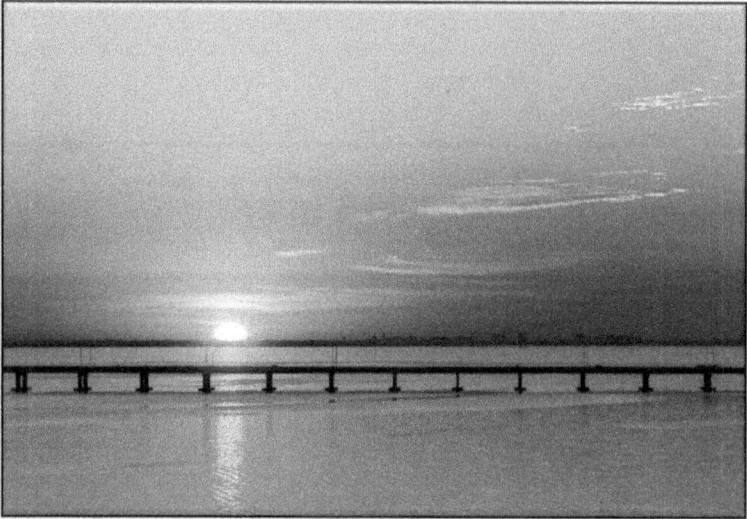

Being Healthy Is More Than Physical Fitness

N ow that we know that the body is not a solo unit but a part of three, we can see health from a different perspective. Our body, soul and spirit are dependent on each other and the Light for survival. Total health means being connected to the Light in body, soul and spirit. So, when we talk about total health, we must also address how to keep our spirit and soul in top shape.

Body Health

Not much to explain here other than being physically fit is what we recognize as a healthy body. Sometimes a healthy body doesn't need to be the picture of a body builder but overall, the standards of what a doctor says we should be aiming for to give us a clean bill of health.

Sleeping and eating healthy contribute to the maintenance of our body and mental health. Our body is a resilient machine and can withstand not having the right maintenance. But if mistreating our body becomes a norm, our body becomes fragile. Finding the time to make sure we properly nurture our body is a must.

Soul/Mental Health

When our mind is alert and our goal is to be healthy, we feed our body to benefit our soul. For example, eating too much candy or drinking too much soda may cause me to lose sleep or not have the right nutrients to feed my body and brain which in return can affect my mental health. Having mental health means I make choices to keep my mind and body strong.

Also, when our soul is healthy, our awareness and perception of ourselves and the world that surrounds us is not tampered. In this healthy state, we recognize that we are not perfect and that is OK. We also realize we do not need perfectionism but contentment and fulfilment for our mind to be at peace. A healthy mind reflects a healthy self-esteem.

Another sign of mental health is my state of emotions being at ease no matter what comes my way. I realize issues will arise in my life and I may fail, but I feel confident that accepting my demise will allow me to find a solution. My emotional state is not a roller coaster but a resource to help me navigate through life.

The last sign of mental health is the decisions I make. They are sound. I find ways to come up with the best outcome possible and I take the time to visualize my different options if needed. In a word, I am "centered" and do what I can to stay at that level that allows me to stay motivated in life.

My mental health reflects my self-love. The healthier my mental health, the stronger my self-love. Embracing who I am, loving life and seeing the obstacles as an opportunity to succeed is the goal of mental health.

Spiritual Health

My human spirit is the "pilot" of my life. When my spirit is charged with positive energy, my spirit is positive, healthy and energetic. I feel empowered to make strong and wise choices that charge my goals and dreams in life. I feel engaged with life and with the people who surround me. I feel I have direction in my life because I am able to visualize my dreams and I understand it is possible to achieve them.

A second sign that my human spirit is healthy, is the knowledge of myself I displayed about me and around me. I am self-confident and show self-esteem. I show self-respect and respect for others. The knowledge of me and my existence makes me happy and hopeful in the future.

The third sign my human spirit is healthy is my liking of myself. I engage with myself and others knowing that I am worthy and do not feel the need to judge myself or others. I desire spending time with myself and others. I enjoy myself and my life and want to be kind to myself and others.

The descriptions above sound like a tall order. Who can maintain and devote themselves to being in that "high" state of mind all day long? Probably not a lot of people. It is a struggle finding time to nurture ourselves.

Being charged with positive energy became a priority to me when I understood my mind wasn't making the right decisions for me and I had a skewed idea of myself. I knew right there the code in my human spirit needed upgrading and I could not do it on my own.

When we recognize that we need to change the thinking in our mind, the desire of acquiring new knowledge is deposited in our spirit and soul. It's like our operating system asking for an upgrade and reboot. An example of this is when I become sad about losing someone dear and close to me. The empty space that this person leaves in my heart is very strong and pulls me into mourning. If this state of sadness is not healed, the pain will eventually become depression. In order to get out of this hole, I need a healthy dose of hope and love in order to move on. This is a vivid example why we need total healing of the body, soul, and spirit.

When our positive energy gets depleted, our body, soul and spirit will come crashing down. We may experience emotional and/or physical pain and we may need healing. Becoming aware of these signs can save us a lot of time, pain and tears.

But help is not available if I am not aware that I need help. I used to ignore the signs and things didn't turn out well for me. It was a painful process to learn that I cannot afford to ignore what depletes my spirit. Ignoring those feelings of uneasiness when I lose my positive energy is a disfavor to myself.

Unfortunately, sometimes when we are young and carefree, we are not aware that attending to spiritual health is important. I know this was my behavior when I was younger. I never thought my body would give up and become sick. I never thought that my mental health would make me weak and afraid. I never thought that my negative outlook on life would steal me of my prosperity. I didn't even notice what was going on inside of me. I didn't even know emotional or spiritual health existed, even less that I needed to tend to them both. I ended up depleting my positive energy so many times that on my way to crashing down, I took people with me and burned a lot of bridges.

When I was a teenager and I heard the words: "I have a broken heart," I did not think anything of it because I wasn't aware of what spiritual and soul pain were. Back then, I had no experience about heartache to understand how the soul and the spirit get depleted and broken. This heartache is not just the romantic kind. A heartache comes when I experience loss, when hope inside of me dies, when something or someone dear to me gets stolen. I felt that kind of heartache when I lost my mother and my father. I also felt it when I got divorced. My heart also ached when I learned about discrimination in the workplace and understood I did not have the leverage for anybody to give me justice.

The heartache also came with a big dose of anger when I was sexually harassed at the workplace and I tried to hold on to my job by ignoring it and at the end I was let go and absolutely nothing happened to the man who did it. When I finally was let go of my job, my former manager asked HR to give bad references of me so I could not get another job anywhere else for a year. All these events left clear emotional prints in my memories. To this day, I still feel the strong emotions in my heart when I think about the loss of my parents, the loss of my belief that I was equal, and the loss of my trust in the system when my workplace assured me they were advocating for a safe environment and it was not so.

Loss and pain are parts of life. Knowing how to repair and heal my soul and spirit will make my life bearable and even exciting and rewarding. Grief is inevitable when I suffer losses. It feels like my heart breaking. It also feels like I've been trespassed and treated unjustly. But for the healing to be total, I must direct my spirit to recharge with positive energy.

The job of the soul (mind, emotions and decision making) when I suffer losses is to find an answer how to heal me and stop the pain I feel. This is how our soul is programmed to behave.

The pain is a sign that I have been wounded and I need to heal. Emotional pain is just like physical pain. The soul will always want to stop the "bleeding."

Understanding what to do when I am faced with losses and pain (physical, emotional or spiritual) is the key to a healthy soul and spirit. Peace of mind, love, hope and happiness (not pleasure) soothe our soul and spirit. Throughout life, I have been in a quest to discover what is the perfect peace, love, hope and happiness that I can retrieve in a moment's notice when the pain shows up at my door. I come back to this answer over and over again, I must refill my spirit with positive energy to find peace, love, hope and happiness.

I used to think that achievements and possessions and being in company of certain people would bring me happiness, and therefore, this would protect me from feeling pain. The truth is that no external possession or person can stop the spiritual and emotional bleeding. I am the only one who can take the steps to healing my heart and my spirit. Doing those things that boost the spirit to dream, hope, and love are the things that bring healing and meaning to my life.

Chapter 6

C.O. Aguirre

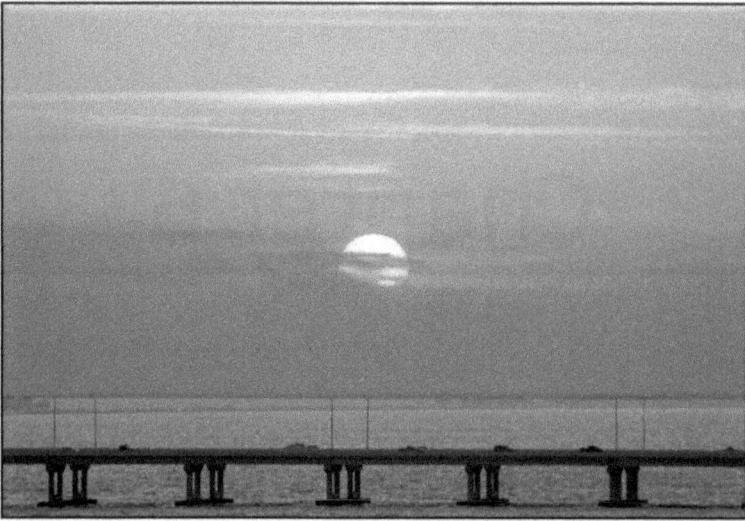

Negative Energy Is Not a Substitute for Positive Energy

W hen life happens, we get emotional. Avoiding emotions like anger or jealousy may be impossible. But when they happen, we must do whatever it takes to cleanse our self from them because they are not a substitute for positive energy. Allowing them in our life may have adverse effects.

Loneliness

Loneliness is a state of mind where a person feels lonely even when they are surrounded by people. Loss and pain can trigger loneliness. According to several scientific studies, there are health risks associated with it. Among them, mental health issues, stress, alcohol and drug abuse, cardiovascular disease, and stroke just to mention a few.

We all need alone time when we are wounded, but those moments alone should be filled with positive energy because if we do not do this, negative energy will just assault the mind and inject negative feelings into it.

Anxiety

In a few words, anxiety is fear of things that have not happened yet. Anxiety triggers the flight-or-fight response causing a lot or hormones to be released. Since the body usually does not return to normal when anxiety starts, the body and mind usually stay in overload affecting the well-being of a person.

According to many scientific studies, anxiety increases cardiovascular disease, weakens the immune system, affects the digestive system and respiratory system, causes depression and other mental issues.

Meditation and prayer can help with clarity of mind and infusing the body, mind, and spirit with positive energy.

Anger

Anger is a natural response when a person feels they have been wronged. But excessive and uncontrolled anger is a problem. It can cause a lot of health problems among them, heart attack, stroke, high blood pressure, digestion problems, headaches, insomnia, and mental health conditions.

Going to a counselor and learning healthy ways of expressing anger is one of the best ways to control it. Meditating is also very helpful to have clarity of mind.

Depression

Depression is considered a medical illness. Its causes are not known yet but there are studies that indicate that genetics, biochemistry, the environment and mental issues may be the cause of it. It manifests by deep feelings of sadness, thoughts of death and suicide, feeling worthless and/or guilty.

It is important to consult a doctor and/or therapist if you think you have the symptoms of depression. It is treatable with medication and psychotherapy.

Other things that help reduce depression symptoms are meditation, exercise and eating healthy.

Shame and guilt

Shame is the emotion that causes a person to feel damaged, flawed and undesired. Shame affects the self-image and self-esteem. Deep-seated shame may cause destructive behavior. Among these behaviors are alcohol and drug abuse, eating disorders, domestic violence, and others. If left untreated, it can affect the mental health and lead to suicidal behavior.

Psychotherapy is a must to learn how to cope with shame. Meditation and learning about loving yourself are essential in the fight to end shame.

Guilt is a negative emotion based on fear where a person feels a heavy load on their shoulders for having done something or failing to do something. Some people use guilt to manipulate others and the one who receives it acts out of fear to remedy the feelings of guilt. Excessive guilt may be an indication of mental issues like depression.

Just as shame, psychotherapy is a must to learn how to cope with guilt. Meditation and loving yourself are important to learn how to end guilt.

Greed

Unfortunately, greed is seen as a good thing in society. It's believed to bring good things like wealth and prosperity. Many psychologists have described greed as an addiction because it comes from deep roots of low self-esteem, anxiety, guilt and shame. Greed is the never-ending selfish desire to have more at the expense of others. The "more" can be money, power, food, fame, attention, etc.

143

People with greed are very good manipulators. And they usually get away with "murder." If you suspect you may have greed, seeking therapy is the first step to healing. Meditating for loving self and peace are important to treat greed.

I also included this section here not only for the people suffering from greed but for the victims of the person suffering from greed. People in power who have issues with greed may never get caught or brought to justice for violating the law or infringing on the rights of others. They may be experienced in manipulating the system. And the more power they accumulate, the harder it may be to bring them to justice. This is a very hard pill to swallow because the most affected people are usually at the bottom of the pole. People who are victimized and feel powerless usually get very emotional allowing anger and fear into their hearts. This anger may end up damaging the body, mind and spirit. Making personal the wrongdoings of the greedy person can cause problems of aggression, mental health conditions and physical health issues. If you are that person feeling victimized, I put this section here for you. Contact your counselor and spiritual mentor for the path to follow. Seeking therapy and practicing meditation are a good starting point. Learning how to let go of the things you cannot control may be a priority to learn and your counselor can guide you through the process.

Self-hatred

Self-hatred is an underlying negative feeling that tells the person he/she is not good enough and not deserving of mercy and love. It is a complex emotion that manifest as inner anger judging and destroying the identity of a person. Self-hatred may be a symptom of depression or more serious personality disorders.

This lack of mercy for oneself, disguises behind the voice of the person feeling the self-hatred. Its purpose is to confuse, judge, beat up, destroy the self-esteem, and take the truth to manipulate it into shame and guilt. This type of negative energy will quickly destroy the identity of the person who carries it.

The best remedy for self-hatred is learning to love yourself. Therapy and meditation are a must to learn how to love oneself. Practicing the positive energy principles will expedite the desire to recognize the negative behavior and getting rid of it.

Loving oneself is the best medicine you can give yourself. It will take away any sadness, loneliness, anxiety, fear, anger, shame or guilt, all the reasons why illness comes into the body, soul and spirit.

Stress

Stress is a form of fear. It may show with worry or with uncertainty or both. In other words, whenever you are in a situation that causes you worry and uncertainty about the future or past, the manifestation will be stress.

Scientific studies show that acute stress may be involved in changing brain function, triggering of disease or aggravating the chances of getting ill.

Stress can give you a jolt of energy but the result of filling your tank with stress is not what you want. Avoid stress. And seek peace to have clarity of mind to make the right decisions.

Worry

Worry is also a form of fear. It manifests as a constant concern about a situation happening in the future or the past. Acute worry becomes anxiety and will develop a series of health issues.

Just like stress, studies show that worry and anxiety trigger a series of mental and physical disorders.

And just like stress, worry masks the jolt of energy it gives you as a good thing. Worry may give you the wrong idea that by chewing worry in your mind all day long will give answers to your fears. Unfortunately, acute worry jumps to anxiety which will cause even more health problems.

Avoid worrying by meditating and taking deep breaths. And just like stress, seek peace to have clarity of mind to make the best decisions.

Jealousy

Jealousy is a passionate emotion based on fear and anger. It is fear because your darkest suspicions become a reality before your eyes (whether they are true or not). And when your mind registers that fear of being jilted your reaction is passionate anger, sometimes to the point of rage. At this point, you may "slay" with words or actions the person who betrayed you and anybody involved with the betrayal.

This type of emotion is so volatile that the energy it gives you may last days or weeks. This type of energy also blinds your rationale and may lead you to do things you would not have done otherwise. You may injure a lot of people when you have an explosion of jealousy.

Besides giving you high blood pressure, jealousy alters the perception of reality affecting your mental health.

When you feel jealousy rise in the seed of your emotions, your gut, disengage from the confrontation, take a walk, take deep breaths, meditate, and pray for peace. Once your peace is back, discuss with your counselor and spiritual mentor for the right path to take. Eradicating the fear of betrayal and low self-esteem is needed to get rid of jealousy. Meditation and self-affirmations can help with this.

Envy

This emotion is also based on fear and anger. The feeling manifests as a resentment (anger) when you perceive someone else's possessions or status in life are better than yours. Overtime, envy becomes anguish (stronger fear) and bitterness (stronger anger).

Just like jealousy, envy alters the perception of reality. Envy may not be an explosive emotion (it could be), but the effects may just be as devastating as jealousy and stress and worry damaging others and oneself. It affects not only physical health but also the mental health and may cause insomnia, cardiovascular diseases, and cancer.

When you feel this envy rise in the seed of your emotions, your gut, break the thinking pattern by disengaging, taking a walk, doing meditation. Ask for peace. When you feel centered again, contact your counselor and spiritual mentor for the path to follow.

The sad part about negative energy is that it's somehow addictive. The payoff for using it gives you the illusion that you get justice and retribution for the wrongs committed against you. But the truth is that the one who gets the short end of the stick is you, not the person who commits the offense. The negative energy in your body, soul and spirit will find a way to destroy you and your health. We do not realize this until it is too late. I know this is true because as a chaplain, I kept hearing that resentment was like a cancer that would take your health away. Knowing this didn't prevent me from holding a grudge against co-workers and former bosses. There were times when I wanted to get rid of resentment when I saw that my blood pressure boiled in a second or when I remembered the wrong committed against me. Still, deep inside of me, I didn't want to let go out of fear that nobody would validate my pain and injury. It was until I humbled myself and surrendered my right to justice that I realized that the way to justice was redemption.

This redemption looked like kindness and forgiveness that brought me peace, hope and love back into my life. And why is it that I have to give up my claim to justice to let forgiveness and kindness be the response for the wrongdoings committed against me? The reason has not been discovered by science yet. But I know that it has to do with the Light's nature.

Fear, anger, shame and any other negative energy cannot produce justice because justice is about balance, peace, and respect. Only the Light knows how to restore balance in the universe. Only the Light can infuse peace into the heart. Only the Light can instill respect into mending fences. Why is the Light the only one who can do these things? Because the Light designed the universe and the Light is the only one who knows how to heal and how to restore what's being broken. And in order to receive justice, we must surrender in faith to the Light. What do we give up by surrendering to the Light? Our ego. What do we gain by surrendering to the Light? Healing, peace, love, hope, forgiveness, and every single good thing that comes from the Light. Is it worth surrendering to the Light? I can tell you that each day I experience life and health feels like a miracle. Life and health are priceless. Surrendering my ego is a small price to have love, peace, and healing in my life. I realize that this is a personal decision and I can tell you that you won't regret it.

Prayer for cleansing negative energy

If you find yourself being overpowered by an emotion fueled by negative energy, and you cannot disengage and leave the scene, a simple quick prayer that you can say under your breath may help you until you are able to meditate and receive peace.

Prayer for cleansing negative energy:

"Light of the World, I thank you for the opportunity to surrender myself. I feel helpless fighting this emotion that is taking over me. I ask that you fill me up with gratitude, peace and love for myself so that I make the right decisions for me at this time of need. Amen."

Chapter 7

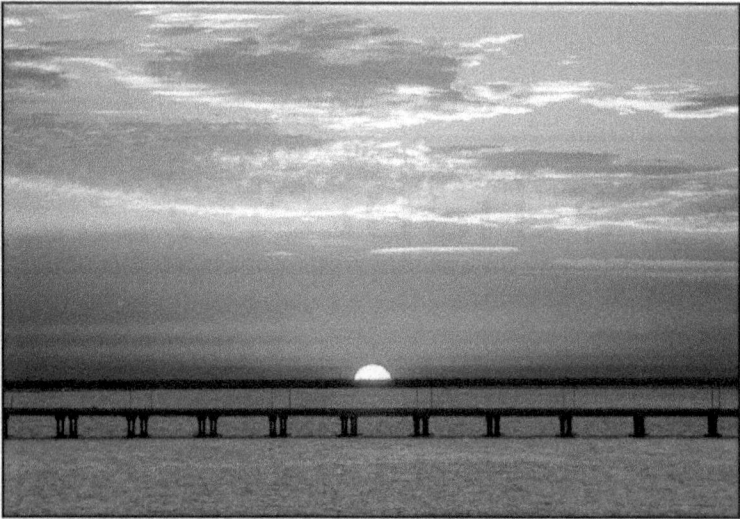

Let's Walk the Walk

Walking with the Light

I didn't know what to expect when my counselor told me I needed to walk the walk. I was at a place where I understood what happened to me in the past and what I needed to do to move on. It was easy talking the talk but when I was challenged to practice what I preached, well that was not something I was happy to do.

Walking with the Light is being connected to positive energy from the moment I open my eyes to the moment I go to sleep. Taking the challenge of getting filled with the Light is one of the most exciting things I have done in my life. It has not been easy but being at peace, and having hope and love are invaluable.

Walking with the Light is knowing that I don't have to live in fear or be angry because connecting with the Light opens my heart to love. And love drives away all fear.

The Light is a fundamental part of me – I am made of Light

One of the most fundamental discoveries and realizations I've had in my healing journey is that I am made out of Light. In fact, we all are. Even though I could feel pain, suffering, defeat, tiredness, hopelessness and hating living, my essence is not that negativity. My essence is Light. There is nothing in me that attaches me to negativity except my filling up my gas tank with negative energy. But when my emotions are triggered by negative energy, I cannot help it but feel like I am the negativity I am feeling. Getting out of this funk can only be done when I align my spirit, soul and body with the Light. Sometimes, this

153

doesn't come natural to me so I must make an extra effort, have a plan and a routine where I purposely fill up my tank with the right fuel that brings the best out of me. Walking with the Light is practicing a spiritual program that helps me understand what I need to do to feed or refuel my spirit and soul with positive energy.

Remembering I am one with the Light

One of the first responses people give me when I want to pray for them is that they do not think that the Light would care for them. Or that the Light is too busy to hear them. Another answer I hear is that the Light is too far away or that they don't think the Light could come close to them.

All these answers could not be further from the truth. The fabric of my life is light and that attaches me to the Light all the days of my life. The electric current that gives me the breath of life, is with me all the days of my life. But if the Light is that close, how come sometimes I feel so empty and disengaged? Pain, suffering and loss will always deplete us of the positive energy that makes us feel content. It is at that moment when I recognize that I have been "hit" that I must remember my direct connection with the Light, recharge and use the tools of gratitude, meditation and prayer to fill me up again.

The Light does not leave me or separates from me. Making sure this knowledge stays with me and I do not get confused about this fact, I must turn on my awareness that the Light is within me. Meditation, observing nature, making a list of four things why I am grateful, and prayer are great ways to keep in mind that I am not separated from the Light. Personally, I like to say a prayer out loud so that my soul or mind can hear what it needs to focus on. The following is a gratitude prayer that I say in the morning and whenever I need it.

Prayer of gratitude for the Light in me:

"Thank you, Light of the World for giving me life today and for your constant companionship. Let my body, soul and spirit be aware of this wonderful gift."

Expressing gratitude every day

Gratitude is a skill that needs to be cultivated when walking through a healing journey. I cannot emphasize enough the necessity to have it. Gratitude is a great catalyst that changes the way we think and do things. Gratitude changes the way we see life and experience life. Gratitude gives a different perspective and because of it, we choose positive energy to fuel us.

It is of the utmost importance that we practice gratitude 24/7 in our healing journey. Of course, there will be times when all we want to do is complain, be angry and indulge in self-pity. Those attitudes for sure bring us energy and make us feel empowered and loved for a minute or two. But usually those moments are followed by shame and guilt.

Now that we know there is another way to deal with life, gratitude is the key to open this new world for us. Why should we settle for a temporary answer and lesser energy when we can have the real thing? This is why gratitude is so important. It will veer us in the right direction when we take the wrong turn.

155

Sometimes we find ourselves not having anything to be grateful for. This is normal at the beginning of developing this skill. One of my mentors gave me a tip. After meditating in the morning, write four reasons why you are grateful that day. And through the day, you can remind yourself the four reasons to be grateful for. After a month of practicing this, it becomes easier and easier to see reasons why we are thankful.

One of the greatest things I have witnessed gratitude do is perform little miracles. Before practicing gratitude, I loved complaining, finding fault in others, being a perfectionist and the list goes on and on. These behaviors blinded me to see the blessings in my life. Once I started to give thanks, I discovered sunrises, sunsets, and friends. But perhaps the best miracle was to discover my skills, abilities, creativity, strength and tenacity. I always thought I was weak. What a pleasant surprise it was to discover that I was quite powerful, and I didn't have to be selfish, controlling, a liar or a backstabber. Gratitude is one of the greatest bléssings in my life.

I am worthy of receiving good things

Guilt and shame are the biggest adversaries when it comes to us feeling worthy of receiving good things, especially healing. In my role as a chaplain praying for the sick, I asked people to visualize their healing. Usually people with guilt and shame have a hard time picturing it. Sometimes they are aware of the thought that makes them feel unworthy of healing. Some other times, they are not aware.

If you are part of the first group and know why you feel unworthy of healing, talk to your counselor, spiritual advisor and spiritual mentor and ask them if you owe any amends to people and if it's feasible to make amends in person.

If you are part of the second group, there may be a deep wound that it is too painful to face now. Ask yourself if you want to be aware. If the answer is no, meditate in the morning about loving yourself. Also, talk to your counselor about it.

If you want to become aware of what may be blocking you, you may repeat this prayer in the morning:

Prayer for awareness of the truth:

"Light of the World, I am grateful for the desire and strength I am receiving to invite healing into my life. Let my body, soul and spirit be open to the truth."

Once you become aware of the truth, talk to your counselor, spiritual advisor and spiritual mentor. Ask them if you owe any amends to people and if it's feasible to make amends in person.

Practicing positive energy

The reason why our day starts requesting positive energy is because if we do not do it, the negative energy will get a foot in the door. Let's remember that meditating and requesting the positive energy principles is an act of love for ourselves.

Every single positive energy principle is needed to maintain our total health. At the beginning you can start practicing one at a time. And as you strengthen and feel confident about each one, you can add to your list until you are able to practice them all. This is the order I recommend you follow:

1- Gratitude
2- Peace
3- Love
4- Hope
5- Kindness
6- Acceptance
7- Inclusion
8- Self-esteem
9- Forgiveness
10- Healing
11- Happiness
12- Self-control
13- Faith
14- Mercy

You can say the following prayer in the morning. Start with "gratitude" only and then keep adding to your prayer.

Prayer #1

"Light of the World, I thank you for this day. I ask that you fill me up with your energy of gratitude, peace, love, hope, kindness, acceptance, inclusion, self-esteem, forgiveness, healing, happiness, self-control, faith and mercy. I thank you for my healing and the opportunity to enjoy my life fully today. Thank you for teaching me how to rid myself of negative energy, especially fear, anger, shame and guilt. May I be kind to myself, to you and to every being I encounter today. Amen."

Walking with my village

Fear will isolate us in ways we are not aware of. It will put ideas in our imagination that we will believe and hinder us from healing. When our mind is full of fear, we may not make the best decisions for ourselves. This is true for every single negative energy that we come across. This is why it's important to build a village that will bring us support and speak truth to all those parts in our mind that are becoming disabled because of the lies we are attaching ourselves to.

Building your village will take time because you must find people that you trust, and you can tell are practicing the positive energy principles. The following are my recommendations of the people you need in your village.

Spiritual community

This is where you find people who practice the positive energy principles. It may be a religious group and/or an intentional community. Make sure that the people you get closest to are as hungry as you are about filling themselves with positive energy.

Unfortunately, sometimes you will find people who practice negative energy in these spiritual communities. My advice is stay away from them. Negative energy is contagious – you will find yourself in a bad place after socializing with them. Remember that your goal is to love yourself and so choose yourself and your positive energy. Love these people by blessing them and disengaging from their negative energy behavior. Be kind and don't judge. We all have been there. But kindness doesn't mean to please them. Kindness means loving them without judging them and disconnecting from their behavior.

Going to counseling and support groups

Behaviors start with a thought in our mind. When we put feeling into this thought, they become reacting. When the thought becomes a recurring action, it forms an algorithm in our brain that becomes behavior. This is why when we chose fear to mandate our behavior, it takes more than wishing fear away to disengage. Going to counseling will help you learn new behaviors. Choosing a counselor that you trust is very important in your healing journey. Ask your friends for recommendations.

Once you have a trustworthy counselor, ask him/her for a recommendation of support groups that will help you as well. Support groups will give you an opportunity to make friends who have the same goals as you, to heal. Support groups are also good to learn new behavior and see spirituality in a new way. Spirituality is not the same as religion. Developing your spirituality will help you learn about meditation and connecting with the Light in a very personal way.

Spiritual mentor

Finding a spiritual mentor may be a task that will take you a few tries. Do not get discourage if you cannot find the right person on the first or second tries.

The most important trait about this person is their record. Are they practicing the positive energy principles? Do they solve problems based on the spiritual principles? You want to know all these things because that is why you want to learn. Having a person with the wisdom to solve issues will make it easier in your health journey.

Spiritual partner

Finding a spiritual partner is like finding a best friend who has the same spiritual goals as you do. They are learning to practice the positive energy principles. You trust them that your confidence will not be betrayed. You can call them at any time when you are struggling, and they will listen. Both of you share your experiences and learn from one another. It may be easier to find this person in your spiritual community or your support groups.

Walking with my commitment

You may feel a lot of enthusiasm at the beginning of your health journey. If this is the case, great start! But as repetition comes unexciting, you may need to be reminded from time to time that you are doing this because you want to respect, love and heal your body, soul and spirit. If you repeat self-affirmations in the morning, you may say this one before you start your meditation:

Affirmation #1

"Today, I am going to love me, respect me and encourage me. Doing my positive energy program makes me accomplish all of these."

Do not numb the pain, heal the wound

It is a natural reaction to want to avoid pain. Who really wants to be in pain? Nobody. When we have a physical wound, we want to get rid of it, so we take care of the wound or we go to a doctor to heal it. Emotional pain is a bit tricky because the wound is not visible and sometimes, we do not know how to heal it. Some wounds were inflicted very early in our childhood and unless someone noticed and gave instructions how to let go of the pain, that wound stays with us and keeps resurfacing to make us aware that it needs healing. If we do not pay attention, we end up feeling depressed, angry, rejected and/or bitter.

How do I know when I am numbing the pain? Having the need to have pleasure without taking responsibility for the consequences is a sign that I am numbing the pain. Running away every time I feel challenged is numbing the pain.

Some of us have tried many things to mitigate the pain without having to look at it. We use substances or behaviors to make us forget about discomfort. It seems like a good idea at the time, but the agony just keeps coming back so we need more to numb the wounds. That action sends a signal to the mind that it is OK to deal with emotional pain this way, so the brain automatically forms an "algorithm" where the body deals with unresolved emotions by numbing the pain. The result is unresolved pain accumulates fear and anger in the soul and spirit and since the pain is not dealt with, we end up with an addiction or addictions in our hands. At the end, we must not only deal with going through the pain but also with having to deal with the addictions.

Ignoring the pain and letting time pass by in hopes that it will go away is not the answer. The reality is that nothing will take away the emotional pain and heal the wound until we face the pain and strip it of the fear and anger and whatever negative energy is attached to it. And the way to heal the wound is to bring it to the Light. What does it mean to bring the wound into the Light? It simply means that I stop ignoring the pain and bring it into the light to look at it. Then, I take responsibility for bringing negative energy into my body, soul and spirit and purge it. Whatever negative energy was attached to the wound (fear, guilt, shame, etc.) I will cleanse it with the truth of the positive energy (love for myself, kindness, peace, hope and forgiveness) so the wound will heal, and I will go back to having peace, love and hope for myself.

After the wound is cleansed, I practice immersing myself into positive energy every day. This is a routine like taking a shower, feeding myself and exercising. Taking care of my soul and spirit are just as important as taking care of my body.

But sometimes it is not easy to stop the addictive behaviors. This is when building a village is most important. Having people around who will motivate me to take care of myself will make the journey easier.

However, having the desire to get well may not be a priority when addictive behavior is present. This is when asking for the willingness to get better is a priority during meditation and prayer time.

Going to a counselor is also important when changing addictive behavior. A counselor will guide me into the right direction to let go of the past and not to fear the future while embracing the present. Having the desire to get well and live in the present are a sign of loving myself.

Learning to deal with people pushing my buttons is the best investment in my mental health. Taking responsibility to block negative energy from getting in me, will give me happiness in life. This happiness is not just moments of pleasure. The happiness that comes from setting myself free of the pain allows me to enjoy life, to dream, to set goals, to see the good in people, to open my heart to love.

Every day when you open your eyes

Every day you get up, the first thing you do is meditate between 10-30 minutes to center yourself. This is important because your spirit needs to be centered and focused to give the right energy to your soul and body to start the day. Just as you need a breakfast to nurture your body, you need meditation and prayer time to feed your spirit.

After your meditation, you may say a prayer like this:

Prayer #1

"Light of the World, I thank you for this day. I ask that you fill me up with your energy of gratitude, peace, love, hope, kindness, acceptance, inclusion, self-esteem, forgiveness, healing, happiness, self-control, and faith. I thank you for my healing and the opportunity to enjoy my life fully today. Thank you for teaching me how to rid myself of negative energy, especially fear, anger, shame and guilt. May I be kind to myself, to you and to every being I encounter today. Amen."

Before you go to sleep

It is impossible not to get "dirty" with negative energy every day. We come in contact with things and people who inadvertently push our buttons. Because of this, we cleanse ourselves from any negative energy before we go to bed.

Getting cleansed is also important because sometimes the negative energy manifests in our dreams causing fear and anxiety. We want to close the door to our dreams before we fall asleep.

Some of the ways we can get cleansed is by meditating, journaling, talking with someone about it, and praying. I prefer to say a prayer, so my soul hears it is time to decompress and go to sleep. You may say the following prayer to do the cleansing:

Prayer #2

"Light of the World, please cleanse me from any resentment, anger, fear, guilt, shame or any negative energy I might have allowed within me today. Help me take responsibility for my behavior that was fueled by negative energy and ask for forgiveness where I owe an apology. Thank you for guarding my dreams and infusing them with all kinds of good things. Thank you for this day and the abundant life I was able to enjoy. Thank you for the gift of myself. I go to sleep now looking forward to waking up with the daylight. Amen"

Take a walk, run or exercise once a day

Our body is an amazing work of engineering. We are so used to it that we sometimes take it for granted. We fail to recognize that it needs maintenance and love.

Understanding that your body needs to keep active is learning to love yourself. Exercising and keeping your body strong is giving it the maintenance it needs. Taking care of your body is a sign of self-respect. And respecting your body is an act of loving self.

Exercising helps maintaining mental fitness and not just physical fitness. Physical activity produces endorphins. These chemicals that act as painkillers help reduce anxiety, stress, and depression.

If it's possible for you to maintain an exercise program, do it. If you are not able to, consider walking. Always consult your physician before starting any physical program.

I always think of exercising as having fun, rather than having to do something that I hate. If you can be active by doing something you enjoy, go for it. One of my friends do her 10K steps a day by walking her dog at the park twice a day. I have another friend who loves bicycling and she enjoys her exercising time riding her bike with other friends. Increase your mental health even more by mixing some fun in your exercising program.

Healthy raw food, lean meats, and non-GMO food

Did you know that seventy percent of your immune system lives in your gut? Even more important, did you know that feeding the right bacteria in your gut increases the strength of your immune system? These questions are important because putting the right food in my mouth can make a big difference in the way my body responds to illness.

The best gift you can give your body every day is to feed it with healthy foods. The less chemicals and processed foods you put in your body, the better. If you are able to eat your vegetables in raw form, that is the best way to feed the right bacteria in your gut. But cooking them is also a great way to enjoy your veggies. Feeding your body with the right food is part of maintaining your body, respecting it, and loving it.

Creating a food plan and following it is an easier way to stick to a healthy diet. Create a food plan and a list of the vegetables, fruits, lean meats and non-GMO foods that you want to have in your diet. This way will make it easier when you go grocery shopping

The reason why I recommend not to have GMO products in your diet is because scientists have not been able to determine how GMO products affect the body. It's better to spend a little more money to make sure that the food you are eating will nurture your body. The same goes with organic food.

In my health journey, I practice the Mediterranean diet that emphasizes greens, olive oil, fish, poultry, beans, and grains. I eat a portion of poultry, one of fish, one of broccoli, one of asparagus, three more of other vegetables, two of grains and two of fruits every day.

Do not forget that your digestive system is your second brain and certain foods may affect your mental health as well as your physical health in a negative way. Sugar is one of these foods. It may give a spike of energy and boost your mood in the short term, but in the long run, sugar is linked to inflammation, depression, anxiety, bloating and dementia. In my health journey, I have stopped eating refined sugar and processed foods altogether.

I cannot highlight enough about eating vegetables and fruits. They will make your body happy, healthier, and stronger. Feeding your body with the right foods is loving yourself.

Take an Arts and Crafts Class

Creativity has a strong healing power because it acts like a channel for positive energy. Scientific studies show that engaging in a creative activity has the same effects on the brain as meditating. It boosts memory, improves cardiovascular health, reduces emotional pain, increases happiness, opens up the spiritual senses to receive positive energy, especially peace of mind. Taking an arts and crafts class also brings a sense of identity and purpose. I cannot think of an activity that will bring more awareness to the surrounding than taking an art class.

As part of my health journey, I have a couple of hobbies that really bring peace and happiness into my life, photography and writing. I especially love journaling because I discover the world around through my eyes when I write.

Allowing creativity into your life is loving yourself because it brings healing, peace, and happiness into your life.

Volunteering

Serving the community and/or my village has also been a miracle maker in my healing journey. Perhaps the most important reason why I volunteer is that it allows me to forget about my sorrows and enables me to see that my life has value and purpose.

Volunteering also increases mental, spiritual and physical health. Besides the benefits mentioned above, volunteering helps with life in general. Some of these benefits are building networks, learning new skills, getting great references, making new friends, and if you are looking for a partner, you may find her/him at that place where you volunteer.

One of the miracles I saw when I started to volunteer was that my loneliness and depression went away. This is how I came to be a healer and met my spiritual mentor.

I had just gotten divorced and I was devastated. I lost my desire to live and really didn't see any reason to move on with my life when my spiritual counselor recommended that I go seek prayer and see if I could volunteer. This non-profit organization gave spiritual support to people who needed prayer. I really didn't want to go but I hated the fact that the emotional pain would not go away so one Friday afternoon, I went. That evening I met my spiritual mentor who prayed for me.

The place was in the back of a rundown building. Walking into the office did not inspire me with great confidence so I did not understand why there was a line of people waiting to get in. But the minute I turned in my application and met the healer, I understood why this place had an appeal. There in front of me stood a man who had the face of compassion, kindness and tolerance. He looked at me and said, "We will get to you shortly. Just sit tight there for a few minutes." I knew right there and then I had come to the right place.

When it was my turn to get prayed for, I came to the small room where the healer was with another couple of people. They prayed for me to be open to receive healing and the blessing of positive energy and to my surprise, this peace came on to me. I went out of this place full of hope that things were going to turn around. I continued to go every Friday because my soul and spirit seemed to love being in this room that inundated me with positive energy.

One Friday evening, one of the volunteers praying for people couldn't make it so the healer asked me if I would want to help. I didn't feel qualified or fit to do it. In fact, I thought, "How can I give something I don't even have?" and I reluctantly said:

"Thank you for asking but I don't think so." I felt the impulse of leaving the place and stood up to go when I saw this woman in line waiting to get prayer. She reminded me of me and how I felt, weak and feeble. The healer then said to me: "Your healing will come sooner if you take the time to help others." I knew right then and there I needed to do this. That's when my journey as a healer started.

In the first six months of praying for people, my depression went away. I cannot pinpoint the day I woke up not feeling sorry for myself. I knew I was freed from it when someone asked me how I was feeling, and I noticed I wasn't lonely or sad anymore.

Now I know I was born to be a healer. And when I say healer, I do not mean it in a mystical way. But rather connecting people with positive energy. My training was not only following the example of my spiritual mentor but also looking at nature and learning from science how to bring positive energy into my human spirit.

Just like some people are born to be entrepreneurs, or problem solvers, or teachers, I was born with the desire to see people get well. I do this by inspiring hope, peace, faith and love for self via prayer, listening and guidance. This comes easily to me and is my way to help people. During the last 10 years I have been a healer, I have witnessed people get well from mental conditions, cancer, heart disease, diabetes, arthritis and others. I do not claim that I did it. I just guided people to find the Light and a way for them to learn how to fill themselves up with positive energy.

When people ask me who heals, my answer is: The Light is the healing source and we all have the ability to self-heal when we are filled with the positive energy of the Light. The only thing I do is guide people to open up to find the healing source and let the self-healing work. I do not preach a certain religion because the Light is not a religion but a reality that we can now see in action through the discoveries of Quantum Physics and science.

I became a chaplain, a life coach, and a spiritual counselor to reach out to people of all creeds and backgrounds. We all need someone to help us lift our spirits up and with gratitude I realize I was born to do just that.

Chapter 8

C.O. Aguirre

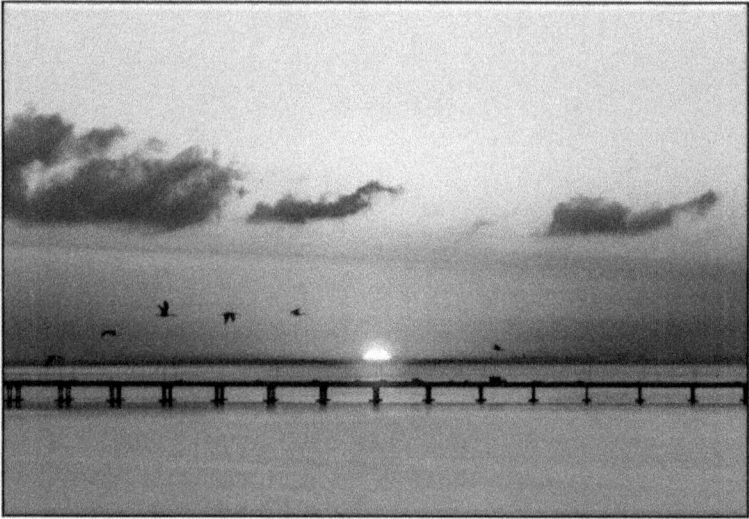

Getting Back on the Horse

I t is really exciting to be empowered and finally realize what you need to do to complete the cycle for total health. For me it felt like I had finally found an answer to the pain I was feeling in my spirit. And even though I knew practicing positive energy would end the effects of negative energy, there were times when instead of wanting to move forward, I ended up going back to where I began. My commitment to loving myself was strong as ever, but to my surprise, I still stumbled and suffered severe setbacks. You will have setbacks in your health journey as well. But when you find yourself there, remember this, setbacks are a blessing in disguise because as you stand up and walk again, you will learn about your character and power within you.

One of the major setbacks I suffered was when I started to become aware that I needed to tend to my spirit. My marriage started to crumble because I felt oppressed in the relationship. I knew my ex was drinking too much and his anger level was getting higher than usual. I reached out to my spiritual community and marriage counselor in hopes that things would get better. For a short period of time, things improved. But it didn't last long.

One evening I came home to encounter my ex-husband in a moment of rage. Nothing I said or did made sense to him. The tension got elevated to the moment when he verbally abused me. It wasn't the first time he had done that, but it was the first time he used words I had confided in him and he took those words and used them against me.

The "fatal blow," as I call it, came when I found out that my ex quit his job because he didn't want to do it any longer. He quit in the spur of the moment without thinking or speaking to me about it. When we were having dinner and told me about it, I wanted to be understanding. I listened to his reasoning, but I had to ask why he couldn't wait to find another job before quitting. His rage flared as if I had committed a crime. He made very clear to me that I was not to question his decisions because he was in charge of the household. I tried to be kind and assertive but firm by making clear that I had a saying in the relationship and the answer I got was totally unexpected. He used my own words of pain that I confided in him about my struggle with being discriminated against to subdue me and control me. He told me that to have an equal relationship I needed to be smart and people of my background didn't have that capability. His raging went on and on with words of profanity and curses, but I stopped listening after he used my pain to make himself feel better.

Once his rage subsided and he felt guilty about what he had done, he apologized and promised me that he didn't mean the words he had used. But something in me was broken and our relationship never went back to that place where I could trust him. I knew at that moment that even though I considered him the love of my life, that wasn't enough for me to trust him with my life. I knew it was over. I tried many times to go back to that place where my home meant peace and love and trust, but I couldn't do it because I never felt safe again under his care.

It took me years and the distance of an ocean between us to be able to speak to my ex-husband again. And when I did, I made amends with him and asked for forgiveness, not because he deserved it, but because I didn't want to carry the resentment and anger in my heart anymore. This resentment only confused me and made my life miserable. It would not let me see that not all men were like him.

It took a great deal of strength and decisiveness to get back on the horse. But once I let go of the resentment, I was pleasantly surprised to see that there were men of all colors and shapes and creeds who were men of honor and respected not only themselves but the women around them.

By letting go of the resentment, I felt that my ability to trust, especially me, was back. I understood that trusting the Light with my safety was more important than keeping myself chained to torturing-negative energy that was sucking the life out of me. And putting my trust in the Light meant that my source of positive energy would never fail me and I could depend on it.

Even though it was very painful, my relationship with my ex taught me a great lesson. When my safety feels threatened or a situation is out of my control and I feel overwhelmed, this causes me high levels of anxiety. And when anxiety attaches to my mind and emotions, it is very hard to go back to having peace of mind. What can I do when I am faced with this situation?

Feeling safe is an act of trust. This is why we feel betrayed and angry against a person or a group of people who break that promise to keep us safe. Rebuilding that trust cannot be done in a matter of seconds to bring our peace of mind back. Neither does it come back by understanding why the other person or group of people did what they did. It takes communication, forgiveness, kindness, and willingness to go back to that place where you can feel safe again. And for all of these things to fall into place, it takes time because you cannot rush your heart to trust again.

When I decided to get back in the game, I started by getting close to my mother. If I was going to have a relationship, I wanted to start by understanding how to love unconditionally. Dropping my expectations of how my mother should love me was a very good place to start. This was one of the most cathartic and heartening experiences I have ever had. I learned that my mother cared for me deeply and her way to show it was not how I expected it. Once we became close, she started to write me letters. Through these letters, I learned about me, her and my family. One of the most curious things I understood was my mom's way of showing love – by cooking and doing laundry.

My mom's letters became the key that open my heart to believe in relationships again. I didn't see her love until I opened my heart to accept her just the way she was. And to my biggest surprise, she wasn't afraid to express her feelings for me in writing. Her beautiful letters are the most amazing love letters I ever received. I am very grateful I had the chance to receive her love for me before she departed from this realm.

After you have been hurt, getting back on the horse becomes an act of faith, trust and love between you and the Light. Faith because you must take a leap of faith into believing that betrayal will not knock you down again even if someone cheats on you. Betrayal will not have the same devastating effect because the love you have for yourself will prevent betrayal from distorting your self-image.

Getting back on the horse takes trust because you are no longer trusting another human being, but you are trusting the

Light and yourself that things happen for a reason. Good things will come out of your experience, even if the wound takes a long time to heal.

Getting back on the horse also takes love because you must love yourself to forgive the other person or group of people. It takes love because you forgive yourself from any guilt, shame, fear and anger you harbored against the other person or group of people. By loving yourself, you will be able to free yourself from any negative energy that may be weighing you down and impeding you from finding peace, hope and happiness in life.

Getting back on your feet is also an act of courage. Life is hard and sometimes doesn't seem fair but staying in the past and having a pity party will not validate your pain. Love and forgiveness will validate not only your pain, but also your existence. Love and forgiveness will open your eyes to see new beginnings. Having the courage to get back on your feet will invigorate you, give you a new perspective in life and open doors to discover your strength, power and impact on yourself and others.

Do not be afraid to get back on the horse. You will be surprised by all the good things that come your way when you have the courage to believe in yourself.

C.O. Aguirre

Chapter 9

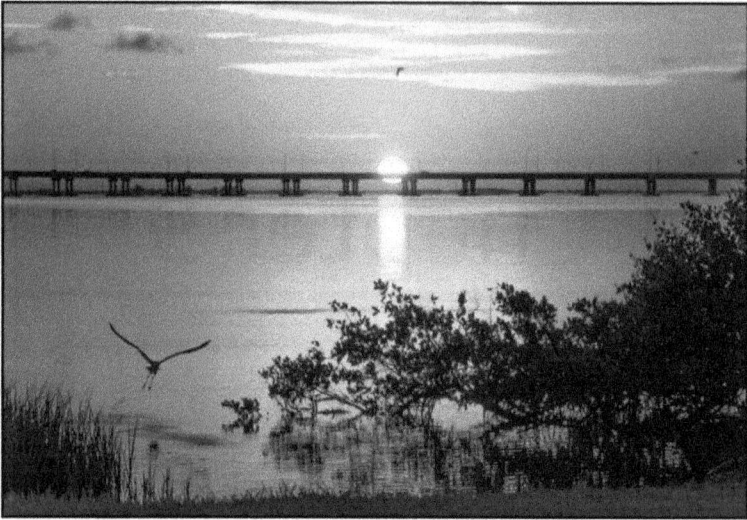

A New Beginning

I have the chance today to start a new life

Today is the only time we have. Yesterday is just a memory. And tomorrow is not here yet. You received today to enjoy and love yourself.

Today marks a new beginning where you get to put into practice filling your tank with positive energy. Today you choose to see life differently. Today you have a new life. Enjoy!

Time to start practicing – you are worth it

If you made it this far, it means you are ready to start practicing what you read. We all deserve to get healing. If you are still hesitating whether or not the Light is interested in your healing, I invite you to look at the sky. Is the sky completely covered with clouds? Is there a heavy storm with lighting and thunder? Is it nighttime and the darkness is deep? Yes, we all have times when the light is hard to find, and it can be scary. But in the end the sunlight appears in the sky.

This amazing light pierces through the clouded sky, the strongest storm, and the deepest darkness. Its goal is to give us sunlight, hope, joy and vitamin D so it breaks all barriers to show up for us. This is how much the Light wants to see you in total health. It will pierce through any sadness, illness, doubt, fear, or anger to give you healing, peace, love, and hope. All the Light wants is for you to raise your eyes to the sky and let it in. I know it because it happened to me.

We all are like the sunrise, full of the beauty and energy of the Light. This beauty is not one type only or designed with only one prototype because this beauty is assembled with multiple elements that make it unique.   The sun, the clouds, the mountains, the city, the water, and the sky become a canvas to create a new force of energy every day. This beauty cannot be put in a box or in a formula because the skies are painted every morning with a new creation to make it unique. This beauty doesn't belong to any human being but brings enjoyment to all those people who take the time to notice it. We human beings are that beauty full of energy, creativity and uniqueness who have the capacity to bring happiness to other human beings. Real beauty is when a person is able to bring peace, hope and love into the spirit of another human being.

Loving life after getting sick was something I didn't think would happen. But I found it when I decided to look at the sunrise every morning and let the Light in. That's when I started recycling my mind, body and spirit. It seemed impossible after having cancer. At first, I felt incomplete, like I was damaged goods. But I couldn't have been more wrong. I still had my body, soul and spirit and what I still had were the parts that had the passionate desire to live.

I know it is true for me that the Light has redesigned me to function more efficiently and with a higher purpose. I have seen it in my friends who are cancer survivors as well. Every day now we fill ourselves with positive energy knowing that it is the best blessing we have received. We lean on the promise that healing, peace, and hope is ours when we fill ourselves with the Light.

I know this is true for you as well. I hope you make that leap of faith and receive and experience this life in abundance that is gently looking at you; inviting you to make the Light the source of your life.

May you be blessed.

Positive Energy Alignment Program

	Activity	Duration	Comments
Morning	Affirmation	1 minute	You may use Affirmation #1
	Meditation	10-30 minutes	You may use a meditation app
	Prayer	5-10 minutes	You may use prayer #1
Evening	Prayer	5-10 minutes	You may use prayer #2
All day	Practice positive energy	Anytime it is needed	Start practicing one each week and increase as the weeks pass: acceptance, gratitude, peace, hope, kindness, inclusion, self-esteem, forgiveness, happiness, self-discipline, faith and healing.
Three times a day	Eat well		Eat lots of vegetables and fruits
Once a day	Exercise	30 min	Walking or practicing physical fitness.
Once a week	Spiritual group		Find a spiritual group and meet with them at least once a week
	Support groups		Find support groups that meet your needs.
	Counselor		Find a good counselor
	Spiritual partner		Find someone who wants to share with you experience, wisdom, love, and hope
	Volunteer		Find an organization where you enjoy helping others
	Take an art or craft class	1 hr.	Find an art class or a craft class where your creativity can be stimulated.

Prayer and affirmation compilation:

The following are the affirmations and prayers in this book. I wanted to keep them all in one place for you to have easy access to them:

Affirmation #1

"Today, I am going to love me, respect me and encourage me. Doing my positive energy program makes me accomplish all of these."

Prayer #1

"Light of the World, I thank you for this day. I ask that you fill me up with your energy of gratitude, peace, love, hope, kindness, acceptance, inclusion, self-esteem, forgiveness, healing, happiness, self-control, faith and mercy. I thank you for my healing and the opportunity to enjoy my life fully today. Thank you for teaching me how to rid myself of negative energy, especially fear, anger, shame and guilt. May I be kind to myself, to you and to every being I encounter today. Amen."

Prayer #2

"Light of the World, please cleanse me from any resentment, anger, fear, guilt, shame or any negative energy I might have allowed within me today. Help me take responsibility for my behavior that was fueled by negative energy and ask for forgiveness where I owe an apology. Thank you for guarding my dreams and infusing them with all kinds of good things. Thank you for this day and the abundant life I was able to enjoy. Thank you for

the gift of myself. I go to sleep now looking forward to waking up with the daylight. Amen."

Prayer for Peace

"Dear Light of the World, please help me be kind, grateful and forgiving. Grant me peace and acceptance of the fact that I cannot change others. And grant me gratitude because you can change my circumstances."

Prayer for cleansing negative energy

"Light of the World, I thank you for the opportunity to surrender myself. I feel helpless fighting this emotion that is taking over me. I ask you that you fill me up with gratitude, peace and love for myself so that I make the right decisions for me at this time of need. Amen."

Prayer of gratitude for the Light in me

"Thank you, Light of the World for giving me life today and for your constant companionship. Let my body, soul and spirit be aware of this wonderful gift."

Prayer for awareness of the truth

"Light of the World, I am grateful for the desire and strength I am receiving to invite healing into my life. Let my body, soul and spirit be open to the truth."

Addendum

A website in the making

I have created a website dedicated to the journey of Total Health and aligning to positive energy. It has excerpts of the book as well as new ideas I want to share with those sharing on this journey.

I plan to start streaming sessions once a week to have meditation time. Please go to the website to get more information:

www.positiveenergyalignment.com

An email to request prayer if you need it

I also have an email address if you need prayer and would like me to send positive energy your way:

Positiveenergyalignment@gmail.com

If you can, try to join the weekly meditations. And do not forget to check the website for more info.

C.O. Aguirre

Notes:

_____

_____

_____

_____

_____

_____

_____

_____

_____

_____

Notes:

_____

_____

_____

_____

_____

_____

_____

_____

_____

_____

Affirmations:

_____

_____

_____

_____

_____

_____

_____

_____

_____

_____

_____

Meditations:

_____

_____

_____

_____

_____

_____

_____

_____

_____

_____

Prayers:

_____

_____

_____

_____

_____

_____

_____

_____

_____

_____

_____

Prayers:

_____

_____

_____

_____

_____

_____

_____

_____

_____

_____

_____

About the Photos

All photos in this book were taken by C.O. Aguirre. This is a collection of sunrises she started in 2017. Back then, she began to notice the dawn early in the morning when she got up to meditate. The sunrises became part of her healing meditations.

All pictures were taken from her window overlooking the Bayside Bridge in Tampa Bay, Florida. On a clear day, Downtown Tampa can be seen in the background of these photos. She also has taken pictures of moonrises that are very remarkable, especially when it is a supermoon. But her favorite photos are the sunrises. They highlight the part of the day when the sun comes up in the morning and paints the skies in beautiful ways. Even though the elements are always the same - sun, sky, water, and bridge - this phenomenon never loses its wow factor because no sunrise is ever the same.

Some of her photos were recently featured at the BBA Gallery in Berlin, Germany, and the Valid World Hall Gallery in Barcelona, Spain.

About the Author

C.O. Aguirre likes to explore and experience life. She is a photographer, producer, professor, writer, and science geek. She earned her bachelor's degree at the University of California, Berkeley. And she received her master's degree at the University of South Florida.

Her work as a photographer was recently featured at the BBA Gallery in Berlin, Germany, and the Valid World Hall Gallery in Barcelona, Spain. Being experienced in the entertainment industry, she has taught at the University of Tampa. These days, she is in the middle of writing and producing a show for children.

She thinks of herself as a modern Renaissance woman because of her curiosity to understand the world around her. But she is most proud of her ability to solve problems creatively. Her goal is to live life to the fullest and help others. One of the ways she helps people is by giving support through healing prayer. She feels being a healer is the most rewarding and important thing she has done in her life.

Just like some people are born to be entrepreneurs, or problem solvers, or teachers, she was born with the desire to see people get well. She does this by inspiring hope, peace, faith, and love for self via meditation, prayer, listening, and guidance. This is her way to help people.

She became a volunteered chaplain to reach people from all creeds and backgrounds because she believes that we all need someone to help us lift our spirits.

And with gratitude in her heart, she surrenders to the realization that she was born to be a spiritual healer.

Read more here:

www.positiveenergyalignment.com

If you need prayer and would like her to send positive energy your way, send an email to:

Positiveenergyalignment@gmail.com

Acknowledgments

A special thank you to all my family and friends who encouraged me to write this book. Words cannot express my gratitude for believing in me.

A very heartfelt appreciation goes to those friends who took time out of their busy lives to read my drafts and give me feedback. I am forever grateful.

And my biggest gratitude goes to the Light for being the source of my life, for the curiosity about life given to me, and for the experiences I have gone through that forged the person I have become. And most importantly, I am thankful for the light that emanates from me. This light has become a reflection of the kindness, peace, hope, and love I have received from the Light and all people who have crossed my life journey.

www.ingramcontent.com/pod-product-compliance
Lightning Source LLC
Chambersburg PA
CBHW061819040426
42447CB00012B/2731